BREAKING
THE
RULES
of Aging

BREAKING
THE
RULES
of Aging

DAVID A. LIPSCHITZ, M.D., Ph.D.

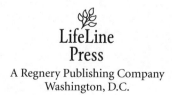

LifeLine
Press
A Regnery Publishing Company
Washington, D.C.

Library of Congress Cataloging-in-Publication data on file. Available upon request.

Published in the United States by
LifeLine Press
A Regnery Publishing Company
One Massachusetts Avenue, NW
Washington, DC 20001

Visit us at www.lifelinepress.com

Distributed to the trade by
National Book Network
4720-A Boston Way
Lanham, MD 20706

Printed on acid-free paper

Manufactured in the United States of America
10 9 8 7 6 5 4 3 2

Books are available in quantity for promotional or premium use. Write to Director of Special Sales, Regnery Publishing, Inc., One Massachusetts Avenue, NW, Washington, DC 20001, for information on discounts and terms or call (202) 216-0600.

The information contained in this book is not a substitute for medical counseling and care. All matters pertaining to your physical health should be supervised by a health care professional.

To My Wife, Frances

Accomplished surgeon, gardener, and, most important,
incredible mother. This book is for you, with all my love
and gratitude for making our lives so rich.

CONTENTS

CHAPTER ONE
Don't Lose Weight!
PAGE 1

The Myths about Weight • Blame Disease, Not Extra Pounds • Why Thin Isn't Healthy • The Fallacy of "Low Fat" • Healthy at 70-Plus • When It's Healthy to Lose Weight • Reversing Weight Loss • When Are You Too Heavy?

CHAPTER TWO
High-Tech Heart Boondoggles
PAGE 31

A Walking Time Bomb? • Unnecessary Surgery? •Angioplasty and Bypass Surgery • The Truth About Treadmill Tests • Save Your Money

ACKNOWLEDGMENTS

I f I have been even modestly successful, it's because of my wonder-ful family. My wife, Frances, to whom I dedicate this book, has for the past 25 years been the major influence in my life. She continues to teach me the importance of integrity, honesty, and of making family a priority. My children from my first marriage, Andrea, Elan, and Howard, have, despite me, matured into accomplished and happy adults. The children I live with today, Riley, Forbes, and Evan, are never-ending sources of joy and happiness. They've made me proud.

My mother has always been my inspiration. She represents the best of what the postretirement years can bring. I can only hope she is proud of her "baby boy," and that she knows that every story about her I tell—and there are many—are written with tremendous love and affection.

I am particularly grateful to my co-writer, Matthew Hoffman, who worked closely with me to ensure that my messages were clear and my words made sense. Without his input, this book would not have been possible. A big tip of the hat to Mike Ward and his staff at LifeLine Press for their confidence, support, and assistance. Ron Goldfarb, my agent, has been a strong supporter and provided me with much helpful advice.

A special thanks to Fred W. Smith, Steve Anderson, and the board of trustees of the Donald W. Reynolds Foundation. It was their magnificent gift that established the Donald W. Reynolds Department of Geriatrics in the College of Medicine at the University of Arkansas for Medical Sciences (UAMS). This program, ranked among the top ten nationally, has provided the clinical, education, and research facilities that have allowed me to explore—and, I hope, thoroughly debunk—the many myths about aging.

I owe a special debt of gratitude to Carole Adornetto, Casey Sanders, and others at the Arkansas Educational Television Network, for their help in making the nationally syndicated PBS series, *Aging Successfully with Doctor David*, such a roaring success.

I have had many mentors and colleagues who have played very important roles in my career. Professors Tom Bothwell, Robert Charlton, and Harry Seftel at the University of the Witwatersrand, Johannesburg, South Africa, are shining examples of superb physicians and teachers. Drs. Clement A. Finch and Jim Cook at the University of Washington, Seattle, true giants in the field of hematology, taught me so much and provided me with the initial research successes that have made the rest of my career possible.

At UAMS, the late Dr. Samuel Goldstein, one of the greatest gerontologic researchers, was my closest friend, confidant, and adviser. Not a day goes by that I do not miss him. Dr. Eugene Towbin, a true pioneer in geriatrics and one of the founders of the field in the United States, did much to spark my interest and help me realize that I could truly make a difference. I cannot say enough about the influence of Dr. Harry Ward.

Until recently the chancellor of UAMS, he is a giant of a man, with broad vision and a talent to build programs. He has almost single-handedly turned UAMS into a world-class institution. Dr. I. Dodd Wilson, who succeeded Dr. Ward as chancellor, has provided me with sage advice, kept me on the right path, and continues to assure the program's growth and success.

How could I not mention my many colleagues in the Donald W. Reynolds Department of Geriatrics? Drs. Sue Griffin, Cornelia Beck, Jeanne Wei, Cathey Powers, Dennis Sullivan, William Evans, Victor Henderson, Pham Liem, Jerry Malott, Ann Riggs, and Ronni Chernoff have provided leadership, direction, and invaluable advice on a daily basis. And Dr. Claudia Beverly, who has worked more closely with me than anyone else and has influenced my thinking greatly.

Finally, a huge thanks to my true mentors, the older friends and patients from whom I have learned so much, and who have demonstrated so elegantly what aging can be at its best. I will always be grateful, and I love you all.

INTRODUCTION

My original plan, when I moved to the United States from Johannesburg in the early 1970s, was to specialize in the treatment of blood and bone disorders. I completed a fellowship in hematology at the University of Washington, Seattle, and later was named director of the Division of Hematology/Oncology at the hospital where I work today. As part of my research, I spent some time looking at the effects of nutrition on aging. A pleasant bonus was that I spent more time with older adults—people for whom the concept of getting older was hardly the abstraction that it tends to be for those in their 30s. Of course, I was getting older myself, and I wasn't sure I liked it. I had a strong personal interest in learning more about how we age, and, more important, what we can do to stay healthy in our 50s and beyond. This is what led me, a few years later, to devote my time to geriatric medicine.

My interest in aging was far from academic. By the time I reached my 50th birthday, I was increasingly preoccupied about my future. Those aches and pains that I used to ignore—and the mild heart attack that took me completely by surprise some years ago—were tangible evidence of my own mortality. For the first time, I realized that retirement—and old age—wasn't all that far in the future.

After my heart attack, I found myself in the novel (for me) position of being a patient rather than a physician. I was almost desperate for reassurance, and even more desperate for information. Before every doctor's visit, I filled pages of my lined yellow pad with comments and questions. There was so much I wanted to know about my immediate and long-term future. How was my heart condition going to affect my sex life? What should I be doing to restore the muscle that seemed to be slipping away? What drugs should I be taking? And on and on. My doctors, polite at first, gradually made it clear that they didn't appreciate my endless questions. I got the distinct impression that they only wanted to talk about my immediate problems—that all of my questions and concerns about the future were a distinct waste of time.

As a patient, I was tremendously frustrated by their dismissive attitudes. But as a physician, the experience proved to be one of those epiphanies that only come along a few times in a career. For the first time, I realized just how much the medical profession short-changes its patients. Doctors are incredibly rushed these days. They don't have time—or won't make time—to truly listen to what people have to say. Instead, they order tests and more tests. It's a lot faster to read a few numbers on a print-out than to sit down and take a really thorough medical history—to ask those endless questions about families, jobs, sex, diet, exercise, and so on.

We've all had the experience of having doctors look at us as bundles of symptoms rather than living, breathing people. I swore to myself that I would never make that mistake. Today, I take whatever time is necessary to answer all of my patients' questions, to anticipate questions they haven't thought to ask, and to give them all the information they need to take good care of themselves. I never, for example, rush them down the hall to the blood lab or x-ray department without taking the time to learn everything I can about their daily lives. Quality care involves a lot more than giving a diagnosis. That merely identifies a disease; it doesn't begin to identify the myriad ways in which patients, with unique lives and circumstances, can protect themselves and stay healthy. Frankly, a good doctor must form a personal connection with patients. If you cannot in your heart bring yourself to truly love them, you don't belong in medicine.

I've now spent more than 20 years in geriatric medicine. As director of the Center on Aging at the University of Arkansas for Medical Sciences, Little Rock, I've come to understand how poorly older patients—those in their 50s, 60s, and beyond—are served by their doctors. My research on aging, and the time I've spent with thousands of patients, have made it abundantly clear that many of our assumptions about aging are, to put it bluntly, wrong.

This has tremendous implications for all of us, those in our 40s as well as those in their 70s and beyond. If you assume—or your doctor tells you—that your memory will inevitably take a powder after retirement, you won't bother doing any of the things that have been proven, time and again, to prevent it. If you're convinced that your sexual performance is on a downward slope, you'll unnecessarily give up one of life's most fulfilling experiences.

I can't begin to count the number of stereotypes and myths about aging that I encounter every day—myths that influence doctors just as much as patients, and which can be devastating to self-esteem as well as long-term health. Here are some of the more egregious examples.

• **Myth: No one should be overweight.** Wrong! Losing weight is about the worst thing for older adults. Even if you're in your 50s and are somewhat pudgy, you'll probably live longer than those rare souls with "perfect" physiques. Want to live longer? Ignore your doctors: After retirement, you want to be a little heavy, not too thin.

• **Myth: Heart tests and treatments will save your life.** Wrong again. There are certainly times when stress tests or procedures for coronary artery disease can make a difference. But guess what? The vast majority of these procedures are performed on people who don't need them— and the procedures can be more dangerous than the disease itself.

• **Myth: Sex and libido invariably head south.** I'm tempted to club any doctor who counsels patients to merely accept "age-related" declines in their sexuality. The truth: Older adults report having better sex than young people. Disease, not age, is what causes declines in libido—and diseases can be treated.

• **Myth: Walking is the perfect exercise for older adults.** This advice is everywhere, and I can't figure out where it started. There's nothing wrong with walking, understand, but what you also need is tough exercise, like lifting weights. Exercise that's easy is exercise that doesn't work. This is just as true in your 30s as it is in your 50s.

• **Myth: We all get weaker and more frail with age.** Well, it's partly true. Older people do have less muscle mass than younger folks. Does it affect their ability to function normally? Not at all. If you stay physically active throughout your life, you'll always be strong enough to do the things you want to do.

I didn't know all this when I started out in geriatric medicine. I bought into the same myths as everyone else, and my early patients were short-changed as a result. Medical myths can have terrible consequences, and yet, doctors who should know better keep promulgating the misinformation they picked up in medical school. They routinely give drugs that have been shown to be hazardous, while at the same time ignoring drugs that have been proven to work. They tell patients that memory loss is normal and fatigue inevitable. They don't talk about sex or sexually transmitted diseases because, as we all know, older people don't have sex. It drives me crazy!

The underlying problem, I think, is that our culture all but worships youth. We have this little voice that tells us that getting old is the same as getting washed up. We almost willfully accept limitations that would never be acceptable in someone in their 40s. Now that I've treated thousands of patients, many of whom are in their 80s and 90s, I finally understand that there's a great deal of life after fuschia hair and navel rings. My patients travel, work, play sports, have sex, go out to dinner, see new movies. They're one of the main contributing forces in the economic engine of our society. One of my patients holds the over-60 world record for running the 1,500 meter. Another, at 75, just earned his doctorate degree. Another, in her 80s, rides a motorcycle. When I see her pulling on her helmet as she leaves my office, I'm reminded that my job isn't merely to prolong her life, but to strengthen the quality of her life. When I wave goodbye, I'm thinking, "You go, girl!"

This two-wheeled octogenarian is the future of this country. Right now, 12 percent of the U.S. population is over age 65. In 20 years, that number will rise to 20 percent. By the year 2020, there will be a 200 percent increase in the percentage of people over age 85. As my teenage son would say, "Yikes!" Policy wonks and politicians have pretty much the same response. They envision a future with failed Social Security because there aren't enough workers per retiree, with crumbling Medicare that falls apart under the weight of all the added patients. These are real concerns and they demand real answers. Me, I don't think the sky is falling, because I've seen a grandmother who rides a motorcycle.

Here's the message I'd really like to hammer home: Forget everything you've ever been told about old age. Frailty and forgetfulness aren't in your future. Or at least, they shouldn't be. The people who lose their independence in their later years are the ones who get sick, usually because they didn't take care of themselves. Age has nothing to do with it.

I'm always amused when families predict dire futures for their aging loved ones. It's almost like they're planning for the day when their grandmas and grandpas get so feeble that they have to be watched all the time, like small children. Sure, it happens. But it's hardly a rule of aging. Whenever I start thinking about all the misinformation about aging, I get a strong mental image of my mother. If anyone has broken every conceivable "rule" of getting older, it has to be her. I do have to keep an eye on her—but not in the way you might think.

My mother, Hanid, lives in Johannesburg, South Africa, where I was born. She's 79 and feisty as hell. Her two-minute history: Her first husband, my father, died young. Her second husband also passed away. So mom married again, and this one ended in divorce. Talk about a triple whammy! Quite a few years ago, I visited her in Johannesburg. One of her best friends, also single, was bemoaning the lack of men. She sounded upset, almost distraught. In my calmest, most-reassuring doctor voice, I tried to calm her. "At your age, many men have passed away...."

"You don't understand," she said. *"They're all with your mother!"*

It turned out Mom was dating two men—one on Tuesdays and Fridays, the other on Wednesdays and Saturdays. Then she met a third fellow, and this one was Love. They've now been together five years and it seems to be working. He's 94, walks two miles a day, and is evidently tough enough to keep up with this fire-breathing woman. One of my nephews, who recently moved in with my mom, told her one night, "Don't worry or wait up for me, I'll be out late." "Worry?" my mom said. "I won't worry about you if you don't worry when I don't come home at all."

I'm relieved that my mother is healthy and happy, not to mention lusty. But I also know that she's getting to the age where things can change quickly. This brings us to what we really know about the elderly. At age 70, the average life expectancy is 16 years. At age 80, it's 10 years. At 90, it's six years. I'm talking about averages. If you're a healthy 79-year-old like my mom, you have a good chance of living to 100 or beyond. That's a long time—plenty long enough to take care of yourself, stay active, and do all the things that you want to do.

Aging does change us, of course. Your body is a lot different in your 70s than it was in your 20s. But with regular checkups and good preventive care, it's relatively easy for adults to stay physically and mentally healthy. Our medical system, unfortunately, deals best with emergencies. You're lucky if you get six minutes with a doctor, and luckier still if the checkup really takes into account your long-term health. The only way that any of us will have a prayer of maintaining our vigor and independence is through prevention.

I spend a great deal of time discussing preventive care with my patients, and I suspect they spend an equal amount of time tuning me out. No one gets excited about routine screenings or preventive lifestyle changes. As my mom likes to say, "David, when I get the urge to exercise,

I lie down and stay there until the urge goes away." I hear this all the time in one way or another. "I'm too old to exercise," "You can't teach an old dog new tricks," "I've been smoking for 50 years and it hasn't killed me yet."

My answer is always the same: You have to take care of your health. Life expectancy is partly controlled by genetics, but lifestyle factors—a lack of exercise, nutritional habits, smoking, and so on—play the greater role. It doesn't matter what you did for the last 50 years. It doesn't matter if you're robust or easily fatigued. It doesn't matter if you hate eggplant or salads. The only way you're going to live a long time, doing all the things you want to do, is to stay healthy. Forget age. It's just a number. But your health, in a very real way, is who you are.

I believe this with every beat of my geriatrician's heart. The healthier you are as a young person, the healthier you'll be when you get older. Get some exercise. Eat well and wisely. While you're at it, keep your mind busy. Take a trip. Go dancing. Visit an art gallery. Above all, break those rules of aging, even if you have to buy a Harley to do it!

Dr. David

August 2002

BREAKING
THE
RULES
of Aging

"I feel so frumpy! I've put on so much weight over the last few years! But my high school reunion is three months away, and I'm determined to lose twenty pounds."   —Margaret, age 55

DON'T LOSE WEIGHT!

Not a day goes by that I don't read a medical study or newspaper or magazine article bemoaning the obesity "epidemic" and chastising Americans for their growing girth. I hear the same thing from my friends, including those who are struggling—and usually failing—to lose weight.

The urge to get slimmer, at least in this country, is almost as common among 70-year-olds as it is among those in their 20s. It's not much of an exaggeration to say that we're all convinced that we're overweight, even when all the evidence says otherwise. Those of us who are thin want to be thinner, and those who are chubby pray for a genuine miracle diet that will finally allow them to succeed when all other approaches have failed. We study weight-loss articles, sign up at expensive health clubs, and worry about every little morsel that passes our lips. We pour billions of dollars into the weight-loss industry—and we've made tycoons of the marketing wizards who take advantage of a vulnerable, insecure, overweight population. They sell us diets that don't work, pills that have little or no effect, and diet plans that usually do more harm than good.

And yet, we keep gaining weight. What's my answer to this?

Quit worrying about it. Carrying around a little extra weight is actually better *for your health than being model-slim.*

I know that's the opposite of the message that a lot of health experts are putting out there, but there are sound scientific reasons—and even more emotional ones—for not agonizing over every added pound.

I'm not saying for a moment that excessive weight is a good thing. Nor would I disagree with the statistics that point out that an ever-increasing percentage of the population is morbidly obese. The Surgeon General recently reported that 35% of Americans are overweight, up from 26% in 1980. Even more alarming is the stunning increase in obesity among our children and grandchildren.

The important concept in the sentences above, one that tends to get glossed over even by doctors who should know better, is "morbid obesity." It's very different from being mildly to moderately overweight. Morbid obesity, which means 70 to 100 pounds overweight, presents all sorts of health risks, from high blood pressure and heart disease to diabetes. But most of us aren't obese. Those 10 or 20 or 30 pounds that cling stubbornly to our middles and backsides are unlikely to cause any health problems at all. Quite the opposite. The research is quite clear that being slightly overweight may have protective effects. In fact, losing too much weight is more likely to threaten your health than having a bit of pleasant padding.

THE MYTHS ABOUT WEIGHT

If you get all of your health information from the mainstream media, or even from the handful of respected medical journals that are read by most doctors, you'd conclude that body fat is among the greatest threats facing Americans today.

In some cases, it probably is. People who are seriously obese die younger and in worse health than those who manage their weight more successfully. But there's another side to the story. A close analysis of decades of medical research suggests—to me and many others—that there's only a modest connection, at best, between health problems and the slight weight gain that tends to occur as we get older.

No one wants to see a country of fat children and teenagers. They tend to be less active than their slimmer peers, and they also have many decades ahead of them in which they're sure to gain more weight and suffer from the resulting problems. But by the time people reach middle age and beyond, moderate amounts of body fat are unlikely to cause much of a problem. Ask yourself this question: If the "obesity epidemic" is causing such harm, why is the American population living longer and healthier than ever? When I get together with my friends—all of us over 50, and none of us in perfect shape—we give each other high fives and proclaim how great we feel.

Here's where much of the misinformation started: About five years ago, a team of top researchers reported the results of a study that looked at 115,000 women. The study purportedly demonstrated that being even moderately overweight was associated with a substantially shortened life expectancy and a much higher risk of disease. This study, more than any other, launched the current war on obesity. In both the popular and medical media, the study was widely cited as "exhibit A" for the claim that fat, quite literally, kills.

Alarm bells should have gone off. This was the *only* report that showed such dramatic effects. In medical science, single studies are always suspect, especially when the findings are at odds with the bodies of research that already exist. Skepticism, in this case, was warranted. In the years since the report first appeared, it has been roundly discredited. The authors' statement that "even mild to moderate overweight is associated with a substantial increase in premature death" is, to put it charitably, a distortion of the data.

But by the time scientists took a hard look at the data and began questioning the conclusions, the damage was done. The war against fat was under way, and doctors and the media trained their big guns at this alleged menace to public health. The same month the study was released, one of the study's authors, in testimony before the Food and Drug Administration, said that the dangers of fat were so great that the agency should approve the diet drug dexfenfluramine, even though laboratory trials had brought the drug's safety into question. The FDA, in other words, was being urged to allow millions of Americans to take a potentially dangerous drug, based in part on a study filled with highly questionable data.

It seems clear to me that the medical profession's obsession with obesity is largely based on flawed interpretations of research, a gullible (and desperate!) overweight public, and the mercantile considerations of the drug and weight-loss industries. Much less attention has been paid to the mass of reputable research that suggests that being pleasantly plump is not harming our health in the least.

Protective Effect?

Here's an example. When scientists look at population data, they find that individuals who are up to 40 pounds above their so-called ideal weights live just as long as those whose weight is closer to the recommended ranges. Research done by Dr. Richard Troiano, now with the Centers for Disease Control and Prevention, has found that only morbid obesity, and not moderate amounts of overweight, significantly shortens life expectancy.

Two large studies—the long-running Framingham study and a population survey called NHANES II (National Health and Nutrition Examination Survey II, 1976–1980)—found a U-shaped survival curve that illustrates the effects of weight on long-term health. People at opposite ends of the U—the very thin as well as the morbidly obese—have higher mortality rates. But what about those in the middle of the U? Weight has very little effect at all. This finding has been observed in numerous studies conducted by researchers around the world. The evidence is compelling, in fact, that people who are 10 to 15% overweight tend to have the lowest mortality rates.

Here's another reason that I almost beg people to quit making themselves miserable about those stubborn pounds. A number of studies suggest that people who are somewhat heavy are less likely to develop some common, and potentially deadly, illnesses. The most important of these is osteoporosis. After age 75, bone loss is a major cause of dependency among the elderly. It contributes to the more than 1.5 million hip fractures annually. Hip fractures are no small thing. They're a major cause of death in the elderly. It's been estimated that more woman die of osteoporosis-related conditions than from cancer of the breast, cervix, and uterus combined. The bones need a certain amount of stress in order to develop protective mass. Men and women who are somewhat overweight exert more daily stress on the bones than those who are thinner. If they also exercise regularly, they're strengthening their bones and providing a hedge against the age-related bone loss that can result in osteoporosis.

Studies also suggest that being overweight may reduce the risk of some cancers, particularly lung cancer. Researchers have traditionally thought that this protective effect might be an illusion—that people who smoke tend to be thin. But both smokers and nonsmokers have a lower risk of cancer when they're heavier. Why this is so remains a mystery.

Even the link between coronary artery disease and weight has come into question. Researchers have found, for example, that the severity of coronary artery disease observed during autopsies can't be linked to body weight. In studies among the living, researchers have examined the insides of the arteries with angiography and failed to find a relationship between the severity of coronary deposits, or atherosclerosis, and weight. One study, in fact, found an inverse relationship between coronary artery disease and body weight. Subjects with the higher body mass indexes tended to have less arterial narrowing.

It's true that some studies have found a link between obesity and coronary artery disease. The majority have not. This includes large epidemiological studies performed in the United States and Europe. Many of these studies have failed to prove a connection between weight and heart disease even after following large groups of people for more than 20 years!

Expanded Waistline Means Expanded Lifetime

One more point about the fallacy of weight-loss absolutism: the notion that virtually every American with a waist larger than a teenage gymnast's should either embark on a serious diet or face the consequences. Think, for a moment, about our parents—the elderly adults who are my patients. A significant percentage of men and women ages 70 and older are overweight. Most of them agonize about their seeming inability to lose weight. But the research is very clear that from age 70 onward, weight and longevity are inversely correlated. In other words, the heavier you are after age 70, the longer you're likely to live. Believe me, that's a hard line to sell! But it's true.

Study after study of older adults has shown that those who are chubbier live longer. This relationship appears to hold true even among the very obese. No one really knows why obesity that's harmful in younger adults helps protect the elderly. It may well be that in evolutionary terms, people who were underweight (or were losing weight) were more likely to get ill or die at an early age than those who were more robust. In other words, being heavy, or at least not losing weight, may confer a survival advantage. But more about this later.

Comparing Apples and Pears

The one weight-related factor that I think does play an important role in health is body-fat distribution. Heavy people who have large thighs and buttocks (the so-called "pear-shaped obesity") are much less prone to disease than those with more upper-body and abdominal fat ("apple-shaped obesity").

Let's look at the pear shape first. Most women, and some men, gain weight in the thighs. The greater the amount of thigh fat, the higher the levels of high-density lipoprotein (HDL), the "good" cholesterol that protects against coronary artery disease. This might be indirectly related to estrogen, a hormone that elevates HDL. But since men with heavy thighs also tend to have higher HDL, the estrogen link is a bit questionable.

Now, the apple shape. Most men, and some women, accumulate weight in the abdomen, the so-called "beer belly." Genetic factors and the hormone testosterone are thought to contribute to abdominal fat deposition. Lifestyle factors such as alcohol consumption and a lack of exercise contribute, too. The greater the amount of belly fat, the higher the levels of total cholesterol—and the greater the amount of low-density lipoprotein (LDL), the "bad" cholesterol that increases the risk of heart attacks. People with large stores of abdominal fat also tend to have low levels of protective HDL. So they get hit from all sides.

For both the "apples" and the "pears," total weight doesn't seem to be a predictor of long-term health. Fat isn't the enemy. Where you put your fat, not how much fat you have, is what determines how healthy you're likely to be.

BLAME DISEASE, NOT EXTRA POUNDS

So if being moderately overweight doesn't reduce life expectancy, how do we explain the fact that most doctors equate excess weight with diabetes, heart disease, hypertension, and cancer?

There's no doubt that obesity plays a role, sometimes a profound role, in these and other chronic illnesses. Yet even those of us who are only slightly overweight have had the unpleasant experience of standing in examining rooms while doctors point judgmental fingers at our middles. Are a few surplus pounds—even 20 or 30 extra pounds—really that dangerous?

I don't think so. A lot of confusion arises from what might be called confounding factors. Yes, overweight people seem to have a higher risk for some diseases, but it's not the weight itself that's to blame, but other factors that may be associated with weight in some cases, but aren't directly related to it.

For example, many people who are overweight have high levels of LDL and total cholesterol, especially if they're also sedentary. No surprise there. The high-fat, high-calorie foods that contribute to weight gain are the same ones that shoot cholesterol levels into the danger zone. If you want to talk about serious risk factors—for heart disease, for example—cholesterol is a big one. It's much more worrisome than a few extra pounds.

Yet we know that a sedentary lifestyle and the consumption of high-fat foods are hardly limited to people who are overweight. Either one of these factors is a stronger predictor of heart disease than overweight. Then there's family history. If your parents or siblings have heart disease, you're at much higher risk of having heart disease yourself.

Hypertension is one of the major risk factors for heart disease, and it's certainly more common in overweight individuals. Once again, however, weight is hardly the only thing that causes it. Age, for example, is strongly predictive of high blood pressure: More than 50% of adults will have elevated blood pressure by age 60. And let's not forget dietary sodium. People who are overweight tend to eat a lot of fast food, processed snacks, and other foods that are loaded with salt as well as fat. The calorie-dense fat component causes weight gain, and the salt can send blood pressure soaring. When you consider that just one fast-food meal can contain an entire day's allotment of fat as well as sodium, it's hardly surprising that so many Americans are at risk for high blood pressure. Ethnicity, emotional stress, lack of exercise, and kidney disease also play key roles in blood pressure risk. Yes, weight is a factor, but I think it's a mistake to single it out over other, equally important factors.

Another factor that's linked to weight is a sedentary lifestyle. Heavy people generally don't get a lot of exercise. That may be why they got heavy in the first place. And once they've put on a few pounds, physical activity gets more difficult. A sedentary lifestyle increases the risk for just about every serious chronic disease you can think of. We know that being overweight is not nearly as important a predictor of heart disease as living a sedentary life. One study, for example, found that deaths from coronary artery disease were three times higher in unfit men at ideal body weights than in overweight men who were physically fit.

Then there's emotional stress. People who don't get regular exercise tend to have high levels of noradrenaline and other stress-related hormones, which have been shown to damage arteries and increase the risk of heart disease and stroke. People who are overweight are particularly prone to stress, along with low self-esteem, because obesity carries such a social stigma. Those who have spent their lives battling excess weight know all too well the feelings of inadequacy and failure that society heaps upon them. No wonder they suffer psychological stress! People who lose weight have an increase in self-esteem—but only as long as they're successful. Once the weight returns, as it so often does, the psychological trauma may even be higher.

It's important to remember that each of these troublesome risk factors may or may not be present in those who are overweight. Confounding variables muddy the water and make things very complicated. Doctors like clarity as much as anyone, and they often fall back on the simplistic, and sometimes inappropriate, conclusion that weight alone is the main culprit.

As far as I can tell, weight is the least of your worries. The risk factors we've discussed, along with such things as smoking, diabetes, or elevated levels of the amino acid homocysteine, are the real things to worry about. This is true whether you're lean as a greyhound or 30 pounds over your optimal weight. But doctors have traditionally confused cause and effect. Because weight is often associated with these other factors, it's taken the brunt of the blame. But as I pointed out earlier, many studies have failed to find an association between heart disease and weight. Nearly all studies have found, however, that heart disease risk is increased three to four times by such things as family history, elevated cholesterol, high blood pressure, and smoking.

I talk to my patients a great deal about lifestyle—a lot more, in fact, than I talk about weight. In terms of longevity and long-term health, weight is probably the least important component. Sure, losing weight can make you feel better, and it might make you healthier in some cases. But the benefits are relatively minor compared with getting control of some of these other factors. Focusing all of your attention on weight loss while ignoring more important lifestyle issues defeats the whole purpose.

Besides, most of the risk factors associated with weight can be readily controlled whether or not you lose weight. Cholesterol and blood pressure, for example, can almost always be lowered into a healthful range with a combination of regular exercise, a healthful diet, and, when necessary, the use of medications. Stress and depression can also be managed with exercise, along with therapy or other treatments.

Of course, the lifestyle modifications I recommend to most of my patients—getting more exercise, eating healthier foods, allowing more time for recreation, and so on—have the added bonus of promoting weight loss. But I rarely make weight the focus. I've found that concentrating too much on weight is more of a distraction than anything else. People get frustrated at the first mention of weight loss. Frankly, their energy would be better spent working on things that they have a more realistic chance of changing—and the things that really matter.

BE HAPPY WITH YOUR BODY

So far, I've talked a lot about the health consequences—or, to be more accurate, the lack of consequences—of being slightly overweight. I think it's worth pausing for a moment to consider one of the less tangible aspects of weight, the issue of body image. It always saddens me when I see the extent to which people judge the value of their lives according to their waist sizes. It's gotten to the point where the only standard for beauty—indeed, the only standard for self-worth—is to be thin, muscular, and fat-free. Most of us will never live up to this ideal. I can't tell you how many of my patients have said that they've spent most of their lives feeling ugly, unloved, embarrassed. Now, that's bad for your health. It's bad for your life.

A close friend of mine typifies this out-of-whack thinking. She's always been a little overweight. She avoids mirrors because she doesn't want to be reminded of how unattractive (in her eyes) she is. For many of the years I've known her, her self-esteem had just about bottomed out.

She eventually met a man whom she loved and married. Her negative body image didn't change, however. She was constantly going on and off diets. She'd lose weight for awhile, then gain it all back. Every year, I watched in despair as she became more and more depressed.

Eventually, she worked up the courage to discuss all of this with her doctor, who referred her to a therapist. To summarize a life in just a few sentences, she made a concerted effort to change the way she thought about herself, her weight, and her life. She discovered that she could look good in clothes even though she would never be thin. Her pleasantly plump body may not have been perfect, she realized, but it was right and natural for her. These days, she's no longer depressed. Her marriage and career improved tremendously. She's also become surprisingly active. She swims, walks, and hikes. She even teaches an aerobics class.

There is a very important message in this story. And it is simple. Be happy with yourself. Recognize your inner and outer beauty. Feel good about yourself, and your self will feel better, dragging you up along with it. Not only will your day-to-day living improve, but so will your health.

WHY THIN ISN'T HEALTHY

Nearly everyone would like to be thinner, and I'd be hard pressed to argue that it's an entirely bad goal. Not necessarily a realistic goal, but one that a lot of us would like to achieve. But stop for a moment. Apart from the sheer dedication that it would take to sport a "six-pack" abdomen or a smaller dress size, there may be some significant costs.

Dr. Reuben Andres is one of the leaders in the field of gerontology, and he also happens to be a good friend of mine. He was one of the first to recognize that people who are moderately overweight tend to live longer and have better health than those who are particularly thin. He was the first to discuss an issue I mentioned earlier, the U-shaped curve that suggests that life expectancy is reduced when people lose weight. Life expectancy is optimal when people are 10 to 15% overweight, and it drops again when they're truly obese. With advancing age, the relationship between mortality and weight becomes less pronounced. After about age 55, the link between obesity and mortality is minimal, and by age 70, the relationship, if anything, reverses.

But back to thinness. The research is clear that underweight individuals have higher mortality rates. Even when factors that can cause weight loss or low body weight, such as smoking or underlying illnesses, are controlled for, thin people simply don't appear to be as healthy as their heavier counterparts. For example, studies in Finland and elsewhere have shown that healthy nonsmokers with a body mass index between 20 and 26—which is within the normal range—have a mortality rate that is 50% higher than those who are heavier. This effect has been demonstrated in numerous research studies that have analyzed disease-rate data from Europe, America, and Australia. Roughly speaking, the rates of death for the very thin and the very obese are two times higher than those who are moderately obese.

We're still not sure what the connection is between thinness and shorter lifespans. There is little evidence that nutritional deficiencies may be involved. Obviously, thin people aren't immune from conditions such as high blood pressure or elevated cholesterol, and they also may be eating diets that are high in fat or other substances that increase their risk of disease. Thin people sometimes smoke, and they are just as likely to have poor health habits as anyone else. And being thin doesn't make you immune from genetic factors that can predispose you to conditions such as heart disease and cancer.

DEVASTATING DIETS

I hope I've made it clear by now that weight alone doesn't make a lot of difference in the long-term health of most people. Losing weight, on the other hand, does make a difference, but not the way you think. The evidence is very clear that dieting is among the least healthy things you can do. Apart from the fact that it rarely works, it's far more likely to cause long-term health problems than the weight ever could.

Researchers who look at large numbers of people have noted that those with a history of weight loss—more specifically, those who lost more than 5% of their original weight—have a higher death rate than those without this history. The important Framingham study, which has followed some of the same people in Framingham, Massachusetts, for close to 50 years, has found that the risk of death in those who lost 5 to 15% of their weight increased from 38% to 66% compared to those with stable weights.

It's not clear why this occurs. Some experts speculate that it wasn't the weight loss that increased mortality, but coexisting medical problems. In other words, people may have lost weight because they were already ill. This would certainly be the case in those suffering from conditions such as cancer or kidney disease. But what about heart disease? *People with a history of weight loss died more frequently of heart disease*, and that's not a condition that's associated with losing weight. So this theory doesn't hold up very well.

Some studies have limited their observations to individuals who have lost weight and have also been carefully screened to exclude those with diseases that might be causing the weight loss. They, too, have a significantly increased risk of dying.

The dangers of weight loss are especially pronounced in those 70 years or older. The evidence has shown unequivocally that people in older age groups who lose weight, even voluntarily, are two or more times more likely to get ill or die than those with stable weights. Above age 75, weight loss is the most powerful predictor of mortality. One of my colleagues, Dr. Dennis Sullivan, who is Director of the Geriatrics Clinic at Little Rock Veterans Hospital, found that hospitalized patients who lost 15% of their weight and failed to gain it back during their recovery had an almost 100% risk of dying the following year. Even in healthy older adults, weight loss increases mortality rates by 40% or more.

Weight loss is very common in older adults. About 10% of those between the ages of 70 and 75 will have lost 5% of their weight; by age 85, more than 20% of apparently healthy adults have lost weight. Mortality rates are lowest in older adults who have maintained their weight. So there appears to be a direct association between weight and longevity in those 85 years or older.

The relationship between mortality and weight is complex. An obvious complicating factor is that older adults have a much higher risk of developing serious illnesses, and one of the first manifestations of illness is weight loss. But the message must be made clear: Except for the seriously obese, dieting is often harmful. The older you are, the more harmful it's likely to be. I always think long and hard before advising older adults to lose weight. There must be a compelling reason for doing so, and the rate of weight loss must be carefully controlled and measured.

One of my favorite patients was a perfectly healthy, rather chubby, 77-year-old lady. One day she told me that she had signed up for a physician-directed weight-loss program, one that used protein powders as meal replacements. She was in excellent health, but she was convinced that she had to lose weight. I did my best to convince her that her weight was just fine, but she still decided to go with the program. And sure enough, she lost 20 pounds in three months.

That's when things started to slip. She gained weight after the initially promising weight loss. She developed high blood pressure, had a heart attack, and was admitted to the hospital with heart failure, and a stroke soon followed.

Fortunately, she recovered. Today, her weight is back to where it was before the diet, and she's reasonably healthy once again. While I cannot prove that her illness and dieting were linked, she sure fits the pattern of diet-induced illness so well described in older people.

Weight Cycling

The risk of dieting is even higher when people lose weight, then quickly gain it back. This familiar pattern is known as weight cycling, and it's extremely hazardous for your health. Studies have shown that men and women who have the greatest fluctuations in weight over ten years or more are 40% more likely to die than those whose weight remains stable.

Losing weight and gaining it back often causes a drop in HDL and a rise in total cholesterol. Blood pressure may creep upward, too. The risk of heart attack, high cholesterol, and other health problems appears to be especially pronounced during the period of weight gain that follows the loss. This might be due to hormonal changes that trigger increases in blood pressure when people suddenly start eating more food. People who eat more also may have rapid increases in sodium consumption, which can raise blood pressure. High blood pressure contributes to arterial damage and is a leading risk factor for heart disease and stroke.

Interestingly, weight cycling is harmful even in those who are young and healthy. In one study, participants went through two cycles of weight loss and weight gain. The results were scary: They lost substantial amounts of muscle mass. Their thyroid concentrations increased. And their blood pressure rose significantly.

If you're dieting to lose weight, weight cycling—and the accompanying health risks—is all but inevitable.

DOOMED TO FAIL

I wouldn't be so critical of dieting if there were even a hint of evidence that it works. While it's not impossible for people to lose weight, it's not easy. The success rate of most, if not all, diets is less than 1%. Think about that. Out of 100 people who try to lose weight, only one will be successful.

Why is it so hard to lose weight? The reasons are complex, but here are the main ones.

When your intake of calories drops, the body's metabolism makes compensatory changes to adjust to reduced food consumption. In other words, there's a decrease in calorie requirements. This makes sense in evolutionary terms because the slowdown in metabolism helped keep people alive during lean times. But it drives modern dieters crazy because the rapid weight loss that occurs during the first few weeks of a diet doesn't last. Quite the opposite. Losing weight becomes agonizingly slow, simply because the body doesn't need as many calories as it did before.

Here's another thing that happens. When you diet, there's a rapid loss of glycogen, a calorie-rich sugar that's stored in muscle. As glycogen levels fall, so does the muscles' water concentration. The water loss can be substantial, adding up to 10 pounds or more in a single week. This explains why diets that severely restrict calories can produce quick and dramatic weight loss. But here's the rub. Glycogen is just as easily replaced as depleted. As soon as you start eating reasonable amounts of food, glycogen and water flood back into the muscles. People really aren't exaggerating when they say things like, "All I had was a great pasta dinner and I gained five pounds." That's the problem with most diets. When you lose weight rapidly, you aren't losing fat. You're losing water. And water is easily replaced.

Everyone has good intentions when they start a diet. But good intentions aren't enough. Most people who start diets don't stick with them very long. Since the metabolism slows quite a bit when you diet, any extra calories that you take in later won't get burned. Rather, they go straight into storage. This means that you'll return to your initial weight very rapidly. It's theoretically possible to maintain weight loss by maintaining the lower calorie intake for the rest of your life. But we all know how difficult this is to do.

Except for those rare individuals with almost superhuman dedication, nearly everyone starts and stops diets, or at least eats more than usual on occasion. In either case, the pounds rapidly come right back. It's discouraging, to be sure. More than that, the cycle of on-again, off-again dieting is terribly hard on the body. Changes in metabolism help explain the failure of most diets, but there are other reasons as well.

The Fallacy of "Low Fat"

Our dietary habits today are very different than they were in the 1950s, when, for example, my mother fed me those delicious marbled steaks two or three times a week. I remember our milk, delivered in glass bottles, having a visible layer of cream on the top. And I just loved that chicken skin!

Of course, we are talking about fat—pure, complete, unadulterated fat. Worse, we are talking about large amounts of animal fats. Back in the '50s, about 35% of total calories in the average American diet were in the form of fat. That's still true today. But the proportions of animal and plant fats have been reversed. Fifty years ago, 60% of the fat we ingested came in the form of animal fats. Today, about 60% of our fat intake arrives in the form of plant fats: salad oils, cooking oils, margarines, and so on.

Animal fats are saturated and are high in cholesterol. Plant fats, on the other hand, are either polyunsaturated or monounsaturated. Animal fats tend to raise cholesterol concentrations and increase the risk of heart disease. Mono- and polyunsaturated fats tend to lower cholesterol and may reduce the risk of heart disease. There's been a real push in recent years toward the plant-based fats. There is good evidence that the decline in animal-fat consumption has contributed to the reduction of deaths from heart attacks and stroke.

Unfortunately, that's not the whole story. The plant-based fats we're pouring into our bodies have some drawbacks of their own. Evidence is emerging that total fat consumption, and the consumption of polyunsaturated fats in particular, may increase the risk of breast, prostate, and colon cancers. For example, a large Swedish study of more than 61,000 women found a strong link between polyunsaturated fat intake and the risk of breast cancer. Similar findings have been shown for other cancers. Plant oils may be better for the heart and arteries, but they appear to be particularly carcinogenic.

When you consider the health implications of eating too much plant or animal fat, and when you remember that dietary fat is a major cause of overweight, it's understandable that more and more Americans are doing everything they can to cut back. We've created an entire low-fat industry. We eat low- or no-fat yogurt, fat-free chips, fat-free cookies, and fat-free salad dressings. Manufacturers have even created fat substitutes—products that are meant to mimic the texture, or "mouth-feel," of fat, but without the calories.

Here's the problem. A low-fat diet is not automatically the same thing as a low-calorie diet. Even though fat has about twice the calories as protein or carbohydrates, it's naturally self-limiting because it rapidly gives a feeling of fullness. Eat a bowl of ice cream or a rich brownie, and you'll see what I mean. It doesn't take a lot before you say "Enough!" But when you eat a lot of carbohydrates, it takes longer to reach that feeling of satisfaction. So you eat more. You might wind up getting more calories even though you're eating low-calorie foods. Of course, this equation is even more likely to add up to weight gain when you top off a high-carbohydrate diet with those little goodies that we all enjoy, like sodas, beer, and snack foods.

The only way a low-fat diet will result in weight loss is if total calorie intake is reduced significantly. This can only be done by restricting carbohydrates as well as fats. So those diets telling you to cut back on fats, but to eat all of the complex carbohydrates (such as pasta, bread, and potatoes) that you want are selling you a bill of goods. Replace fat calories with carbohydrate calories, and your weight will stay the same. Replace fat calories with even greater amounts of carbohydrate calories, and guess what? Your weight will increase.

Our sedentary lifestyles don't help, of course. We spend a lot of time in front of the television, and research has shown that that is one of the highest-calorie zones in the house. So despite our attempts to eat healthier foods, we're actually eating as much fat as we ever did. We're taking in more calories from low-fat foods, and our overall calorie intakes are way up.

HEALTHY AT 70-PLUS

Many of my patients' children are nearly frantic about their parents' weight. I suspect that this is partly because they're so concerned about their own weight that they project their feelings onto their parents. Or maybe it's because they blame body fat for causing declines in energy or activity levels. I'm sure it's also because they believe, like most Americans, that those few extra pounds will lead their parents straight into the arms of a heart attack or stroke.

My advice, once again, is to relax. All of my patients are elderly, and the vast majority have struggled with weight throughout their lives. It's not exactly a new issue for them. Frankly, anyone who has made it to age 75 or 80 without losing weight is unlikely to make dramatic changes at that point.

Nor, I might add, should they want to. As I pointed out earlier, there's good evidence that beyond the age of 70, it's better to have a little too much weight than too little. In fact, losing weight at that age is likely to be a problem because losing weight or having a low body weight carries a poor prognosis. Being overweight definitely does not shorten life in this age group, and it may be beneficial.

In our thin-obsessed society, it's easy to ignore the obvious: The vast majority of people 70 years and older are not willowy reeds. Nature's plan, as far as I can see, is for older people to get a little bit heavy. Heavy, as we've seen, means a longer life.

Weight is not constant. From age 30 to about 65, we all tend to gain weight. After that, weight tends to stabilize. Then, after 75, the weight tends to fall off. We all know this by looking at the people around us. This is the way it was meant to be. Weight by itself does not seem to contribute significantly to the diseases that afflict us in late life.

Please, take my advice. If your parents are getting up in years, or if you're 70-plus yourself, don't struggle to lose weight. Don't! I've been giving this advice for years, and I'm still amazed by the number of people who either ignore me entirely, or misinterpret what I said. Just yesterday, an irate daughter came to see me. She said that she was shocked that I'd told her mother, who's a little on the plump side, to ignore nutritional advice and eat anything she wanted. I said no such thing!

What I did tell her mother was that her weight was fine. Since she wasn't morbidly obese, and since her overall health was good, I saw no reason to make any changes. I certainly wouldn't want her to gain more weight, or to take my advice as an invitation to go on a feeding frenzy. But I also didn't want her to feel pressured to lose weight, just because our society—or her family—thought she should.

As a geriatrician, one of the most serious problems I see in older adults is losing weight. I know that sounds strange, but it's true. It's simply not natural for older adults to start losing weight. If they do, I know that their risk of illness is going to rise—or that something's already happening that's causing them to eat less or absorb fewer nutrients. In this age group, losing any amount of weight is likely to have serious consequences.

Here's one example. Advancing age is invariably accompanied by a loss of muscle. In fact the average 70-year-old has about half the muscle that he or she had at age 40. Muscle is the most metabolically active tissue in the body. Most of the body's energy or calorie needs are determined by muscle mass. Less muscle mass means lower calorie needs, which in turn means less food intake.

Okay, let's see how this plays out. The average 80-year-old consumes a third fewer calories than he or she did earlier in life. This is where problems start to develop. They may need fewer calories, but their need for essential nutrients, with the exception of carbohydrates, doesn't change at all. If anything, their daily need for protein and most vitamins and minerals may increase slightly.

Let's put this in perspective. The average 20-year-old requires 0.8 gram of protein per kilogram of body weight. The average 75- to 90-year-old requires 1.0 gram. Since total food intake is reduced by a third in older persons, it follows that their intake of protein and essential vitamins and minerals is also reduced by a third. You can see where this is going. All adults ages 70 and older have a very high risk of nutritional deficiencies—a risk that's exacerbated by their increased likelihood for having a serious illness.

So you can see why I get worried when older adults start losing weight. I also worry when the weight loss is deliberate. They may feel as though it's healthy to slim down, but they simply don't have the nutritional reserves to permit it. My feeling is that any older adult who has lost 5% or more of his or her original weight should see a doctor right away. And they certainly shouldn't put themselves at risk with needless dieting.

When It's Healthy to Lose Weight

There are a few exceptions to all of this. There are times when I do advise older people to lose weight—but there must be good medical reasons for doing so. For example:

High blood pressure. Many Americans ages 70 and older who are overweight have high blood pressure. Most of them can lower blood pressure without the need for medications just by restricting salt intake and losing a very modest amount of weight. The usual advice is for people to lose no more than 5 to 10% of their weight over six months to a year. The combination of modest weight loss with healthier diets and exercise is usually enough to improve blood pressure.

Diabetes. This is probably the main reason I'd advise people, including those over the age of 70, to lose weight. In type 2 diabetes, obesity reduces the ability of insulin to transport glucose into cells. People who lose as little as 5 to 10% of their weight often have a great improvement in blood glucose levels, and a reduced need for medications. Weight loss can also help reduce the medical problems that often accompany diabetes, such as nerve damage or blindness.

Osteoarthritis. People who carry extra weight commonly experience back, hip, or knee pain. Once again, losing as little as a few pounds can lead to marked improvements.

Breathing problems. A condition called sleep apnea, in which breathing periodically stops during sleep, is almost always accompanied by excessive weight. People who lose weight will find that their air passages stay open more readily at night. They'll also snore less, and have less of the daytime fatigue that results from interrupted sleep.

There are other medical reasons why I might advise an elderly patient to lose weight, but these are the main ones. The one thing I'd never do is send them off with a few pamphlets and leave them to sort out the diet on their own. That's safe, if ineffective, for younger adults, but people 70 and older who need to lose weight should do so under a doctor's supervision, both to prevent possible nutritional deficiencies and to ensure that the weight stays off rather than cycling up and down in destructive ways.

REVERSING WEIGHT LOSS

When one of my patients is losing weight without trying to, I want to know why. The reasons are usually pretty obvious. Except in those cases when people have serious underlying illnesses, the problem is usually as simple as consuming too few calories. The body responds by breaking down fat as well as muscle to get the energy it needs. This is what causes weight loss—and it also contributes to the progressive loss of strength and coordination that I often see in older adults. Forget the issue of weight for a moment. Falls and fractured bones are among the leading cause of age-related physical declines, and they're largely caused by a reduction in muscle strength.

How do you preserve healthy fat and muscle reserves when older folks are losing weight? The main approach is to customize a diet that's high in protein and calories, yet low in "empty," or non-nutritious, calories. Older adults need large amounts of protein, especially because they're more likely to have other health conditions that require a greater intake of this important nutrient. It sounds simple, but getting someone to eat when they don't have a robust appetite is a challenge. What I often tell my patients is, "If it's bad for you, eat it!" I know, this may seem to con- tradict what I said earlier about the importance of maintaining a nutri- tious diet. In this case, however, it makes sense. I want people to really fill up on the kinds of foods they might have avoided when they were younger. Especially foods that are high in fat because fat, with 9 calories per gram, is the most concentrated source of energy.

Bacon and eggs are good. So are red meat, fried fish, and fried chicken. Don't take off that delicious chicken skin! Throw out the yogurt and bring in high-fat ice cream. Don't bother with sodas and candy; they provide calories, but are devoid of useful protein or fat. However, choco- late is a good choice because it's rich in fat and protein. I often recom- mend milkshakes because most people like them, and they're easy to eat even when you're not especially hungry.

I must tell you about one of my patients, who, at age 80, developed heart disease. His wife was totally convinced that the only way to save his life was to lower his fat intake. She was a hard taskmaster, and she made it her life's goal to remove every vestige of fat from his diet. Cereal for breakfast, broccoli and chicken for lunch, and chicken and broccoli for dinner. I am not sure what happened to his cholesterol, but boy, did he lose weight. In three months, he dropped from 150 to 110 pounds. His strength dropped to nothing, and he was ultimately unable to walk.

He was referred to me by another physician, who suspected that his rapid decline may have been due to some kind of stroke. It didn't take long to recognize what was happening. The poor man was starving to death. I insisted that his wife loosen up. "Let him eat anything he wants," I told her. Once he started eating normally, and with the help of exercise and physical therapy, he came back around. Today, he remains eternally grateful, his wife is contrite, and for the first time in more than sixty years of marriage he seems to have the upper hand in making decisions. A happy ending to a potentially tragic story!

So here's the bottom line. Don't worry too much about weight once you or your loved ones hit that 70th birthday. You don't want to be obese, but you don't want to be thin, either. Worry instead about staying healthy, eating well, and exercising regularly. If you do these few things, you're going to feel better and stay healthier, regardless of what number you see when you stand on the scale.

WHEN ARE YOU TOO HEAVY?

Because I'm a geriatrician, all of my patients are elderly—the ones for whom any amount of weight loss is cause for concern. I mention this because I don't want to give the impression that I think it's acceptable for everyone to walk around with enormous amounts of weight. If you're pleasantly plump, I salute you! But some of us, regrettably, carry around a lot more padding than we need. A little weight is good for you. Too much causes all sorts of problems.

I said earlier than no one has conclusively shown that modest amounts of extra weight are significant risk factors for heart disease, stroke, or other serious health threats. The rules change, however, when we're talking about serious obesity. That's where the link between weight and longevity is strongly established. To put it simply, people who are massively obese aren't going to live as long as those who are just a little plump. They're going to have a lot more health problems. Their social lives may suffer because they can't get around very well. They're more likely to have trouble sleeping. Even working in the yard or playing with children may cause them discomfort.

In medical terms, "morbid obesity" means that someone is 70 to 100 or more pounds overweight. That's a lot, and it's dangerous. Lesser amounts of weight aren't as serious, but they aren't necessarily benign, either.

How can you tell if you're in the "pleasantly plump" or "morbidly obese" categories?

It's a little tricky. For starters, your weight is determined by your height and body composition. Thin-boned and slight individuals have lower weight thresholds than those who are big-boned. It's entirely possible for a large woman to weigh 160 or 170 pounds and still be within a reasonable weight. Conversely, a small woman who weighs 140 might be obese.

The way we work this out is by using a measure called the body mass index, or BMI. It gives a number that isn't influenced by your body frame. Thus, someone with a BMI of 19 to 24 is considered to be normal weight, regardless of the number they see on the bathroom scale.

I'm not big on math problems, but the BMI is easy enough to figure out on your own.

- Convert your weight to kilograms. There are 2.2 pounds per kilogram. So if you weigh 132 pounds, divide it by 2.2 to get 60 kilograms.
- Convert your height to meters. One meter is 39.37 inches. If you're 65 inches tall, divide it by 39.37 to get 1.65 meters.
- Divide your weight (60 kilograms) by your height, squared (1.65 ×1.65). This is your BMI—in this case, 22.03.

Again, BMI of 19 to 24 is normal. Grade 1 obesity, the mildest form, is a BMI between 25 and 29. Grade 2 obesity is 29 and 35. Morbid obesity, the most serious form, is a BMI above 40.

The vast majority of Americans have grade 1 and 2 obesity. It means they can be up to a third over their ideal weights. I refer to them as "pleasantly plump" or "a little overweight." This much extra weight isn't necessarily ideal, but it's unlikely to be harmful, either. Those who are morbidly obese, on the other hand, need to take it seriously and work with their doctors to come up with a sensible weight-loss plan.

You already know how I feel about diets. I despise them because of the underlying assumption that people can just eat less for awhile, maybe get some exercise, and watch the weight fall away. Well, guess what? The weight is going to come right back. Diets by definition are a short-term process. That can't work for those who really need to lose weight. People have to change their entire eating style, not for a month or a year, but for the rest of their lives.

There are all sorts of sensible eating plans out there. The government's Food Guide Pyramid, to take one example, concisely displays all of the information you will ever need to achieve a balanced diet. But how many of us measure out our foods in grams and ounces? How many of us want to be bothered figuring out a complex chart?

Smart eating doesn't have to be that complicated. Basically, here's what it comes down to.

1. **Eat three sensible meals a day.** Add a midmorning and mid-afternoon snack. Forget about skipping meals, especially breakfast. Studies show that people who skip meals are *more* likely to gain weight.

2. **Don't rush when you eat.** You'll take in more calories than you will by eating slowly. The reason: It takes the stomach fifteen to twenty minutes to send "full" signals to the brain. If you shovel it in with both hands, you'll overload the stomach before it has a chance to say "No more."

3. **Keep your diet balanced.** That means getting a reasonable amount of protein, carbohydrate, and, yes, fat. Forget the calculations. We all know what "reasonable" means. A balanced diet will help you feel satisfied at reasonable caloric intakes.

4. **Watch portion sizes.** A plateful of French fries is too many. As a general rule, with the exception of salads, if a portion of any food fills more than a quarter of your plate, you're taking too much.

5. **Eat similar meals on most days of the week.** True, variety is the spice of life, but consistency makes it easier to achieve dietary balance.

6. **Eat out only once or twice a week.** I know, it's tough when you're working long hours. Fast-food restaurants do make our lives easier. But resist them. You'll easily get more fat or calories in a single take-out meal than you should get in an entire day.

7. **Give up the snacks.** For many of us, this is the biggest obstacle to a successful nutritional future. We all like to snack. It fills us up between meals. It's a great way to avoid doing work. And it makes

us feel good. But it has to be done. No matter how many promises you make to eat "just one," it never seems to work that way. For me, one cookie is never enough. One invariably turns into ten—or, on many occasions, the entire package. Better not to get started in the first place.

CHAPTER TWO

"I had to have a physical for my new job. I was feeling pretty good, I guess, but one of the tests showed I had some blockage in my arteries, so they scheduled me for this angioplasty next week. They said I'll be able to start back to work in about four weeks." —*Milton, age 63*

HIGH-TECH HEART BOONDOGGLES

The American health care system has the expertise and technical savvy to diagnose more conditions and create more innovative treatments than the rest of the world combined. Our surgeons, radiologists, and other specialists can almost literally bring people back from death's door. Heart pumps that promise to work as well as or better than transplants. High-powered vaccines. Robot-controlled surgery. And our medical successes just keep on coming.

This is especially true when it comes to the heart. Cardiologists have the tools and ability to get things done—along with the attitude that doing something is almost always better than doing nothing. Cardiologists and cardiac surgeons approach blocked coronary arteries in much the way a mechanic approaches a blocked gas line in a car: "Gotta open it up, maybe tear it out and replace it."

Gotta open it up? *Angioplasty.* Tear it out and replace it? *Bypass surgery.*

Let me warn you right now: Most cardiologists will talk you into angioplasty or bypass surgery if you let them. Blockages or narrowing in the coronary arteries are never good things, but neither should they automatically put you first in line for the operating suite. Surgeons, remember, have this thing about blockages. If a blood vessel is supposed to be wide open and it's not, they're likely going to want to widen it, regardless of symptoms.

But get this: In more than 60% of cases like this, heart attacks are caused by blockages in blood vessels that appeared normal during angiograms. They're not caused by the blood vessels that triggered all the concern in the first place. Combine that with very high risks for developing a serious, potentially life-threatening infection after surgery, and an equally high risk for sustaining irreversible cognitive declines. In other words, the operation might be a success, but you could die anyway.

A WALKING TIME BOMB?

Heart health is one of the areas of medicine that older Americans, and the baby boomers just behind them, should approach with extreme caution. There's an epidemic of coronary artery disease in this country. Doctors have responded with a battery of invasive procedures—procedures that haven't necessarily been shown to be necessary, and which, in some cases, can do more harm than good.

Here's a story that should cause anyone, surgeons and patients alike, to think twice before entering the operating room. One of my patients, a remarkably healthy 78-year-old, vacations in Europe every year. To make sure that everything's ticking along the way it should, he always schedules a treadmill stress test before he goes out of town. Three years ago, for the first time, the results of the test were abnormal. So his doctor did an angiogram. Radioactive dye is injected through a catheter into the coronary arteries in order to detect blockages that can prevent adequate blood from reaching the heart. The angiogram showed that three coronary arteries were severely narrowed. The next day, he underwent coronary bypass surgery.

The surgery went well. When I visited him a few weeks afterward, he couldn't quit praising the cardiologist and surgeon. "I was a walking time bomb," he kept saying. "Thank God they found it in time." A year later, the picture wasn't so rosy. His heart continued to do fine, but his memory had deteriorated severely—so much so that he struggled to remember people's names or what he'd done a few minutes before. Profound memory loss is a well-recognized complication of bypass surgery. Doctors consider it an acceptable tradeoff for a presumably lifesaving procedure.

But did this elderly man, who was not only robust before the procedure, but didn't even have heart symptoms, really need the surgery? The answer, as I'll show in the following pages, is no. There is no evidence—and I mean *none*—that surgery for patients like this prolongs life or reduces the risk of heart attacks. Yes, surgery can reduce chest pain, breathlessness, or other symptoms, but this man had no symptoms! And when you consider that the risk of cognitive impairment following coronary bypass surgery approaches 40%, I can't imagine why his doctors went ahead with it. A lot of elderly patients have Alzheimer's disease or other forms of dementia. They can't afford additional memory loss, certainly not for a procedure with questionable benefits and uncertain outcomes.

Here's a bit of perspective. The heart is like an engine that never stops. It's constantly taking blood in and pumping it out. Obviously, the arteries that carry blood, oxygen, and nutrients to the heart have to be healthy for the heart to survive. Blood flow is so important that Nature, as it often does, created redundant systems. If the coronary arteries become too narrow to carry sufficient amounts of blood, the heart can form secondary, or collateral, blood vessels that bypass the damaged sections. This means that the heart may get enough blood even when the main pipes are somewhat blocked.

Cardiologists sometimes disregard this possibility. Once diagnostic tests reveal that one or more of the coronary arteries is narrowed, they feel almost compelled to go in and do something, whether the heart is getting enough blood or not. It's not that this attitude is entirely wrong. There's no question that people with narrowed coronary arteries have an elevated risk of heart attack. But as I said earlier, in more than half of these types of blockages, heart attacks occur because of blockages in blood vessels that looked fine on the angiogram, and *not* in the blood vessels that triggered all the concern in the first place.

There are times when surgery or other procedures are needed to restore normal blood flow to the heart. I'll discuss them in some detail later because I think it's critical for patients to understand the circumstances that may demand surgery, as well as the circumstances that don't.

A LOOK AT CORONARY ARTERY DISEASE

Coronary artery disease, heart attacks, and heart failure are far and away the leading causes of death in the United States. In 1998, according to the Centers for Disease Control and Prevention, more than 1.1 million people had a heart attack. In the same year, coronary artery disease killed 403,000 people. Things are going to get worse because Americans are getting older, and the rate of coronary artery disease increases sharply with age. In relatively young people, ages 55 to 64, the rate of coronary artery disease is 181 per 100,000 people. The incidence jumps to 1,252 in the decade beginning at age 75, and to 3,743 after age 85. Diseases of the heart and arteries account for 41% of all deaths in the United States.

Let me back up for a moment to explain what coronary artery disease is. It starts with atherosclerosis, deposits of fat and cholesterol that accumulate in the arteries that carry blood to the heart. The deposits, which look like fatty streaks, start at a very young age. Autopsies have shown that 60% of those in their 20s have some degree of atherosclerosis. Over time, the deposits get thicker as well as harder. The hardening sludge, known as arterial plaque, prevents the arteries from contracting and relaxing the way they should—hence the other term for this condition: "hardening of the arteries." It also narrows the inside opening of blood vessels and reduces the amount of blood that gets through.

On occasion, severe plaque buildups cause sharp chest pains, or angina. This tends to occur during exercise, when the heart needs more blood than the narrowed arteries can supply. More seriously, the hard outer coating of the plaques can rupture, allowing the softer fat underneath to squeeze out and potentially jam a blood vessel. Clots also tend to form in the plaque-filled, damaged portions of arteries. These clots are a major cause of heart attacks.

Many, many things contribute to atherosclerosis and coronary artery disease. One of the main ones is diet. People who eat a lot of saturated fat tend to have high levels of cholesterol in the blood. More specifically, they have elevated levels of low-density lipoprotein (LDL), the type of cholesterol that adheres to artery walls, and low levels of high-density lipoprotein (HDL), the protective type of cholesterol that removes LDL from the blood. The risk of having a heart attack is greatly increased when your LDL is high and your HDL is low—the usual consequences of eating a high-fat, low-fiber diet. Elevated cholesterol can also be due to genetic factors; in these cases, controlling diet won't make much of a difference. Unless cholesterol is lowered with medication, the risk of having a heart attack at a young age is greatly increased.

You're much more likely to get coronary artery disease if your parents, siblings, or other close relatives have it. Men get coronary artery disease more than women. Smoking can cause it. So can high blood pressure, diabetes, and persistent emotional stress. An amino acid called homocysteine, which tends to be elevated in those who have low levels of vitamin B12 and folic acid in their bodies, is a very strong predictor of coronary artery disease.

The growing awareness of these and other coronary artery disease risk factors has resulted in a significant reduction in heart attacks (coronary artery disease, however, is still on the rise). Men and women today are 34% less likely to have heart attacks than they were a few decades ago. Part of the reason, of course, is that more and more people are doing the sensible things: not smoking, eating better, and so on. What about advances in medical intervention and surgery? Well, they've helped, but not as much as you might think. Studies suggest that they may have reduced the risk of dying from heart disease between 1 and 5%. Early diagnosis and rapid access to emergency medical care may account for 10% of the improved outcomes. Lifestyle factors play the greater role.

Arterial Blockages

Let's return to the issue I raised earlier—that arterial blockages by themselves are rarely an indication for surgery. First of all, many people have these blockages. A study reported in the *American Journal of Medicine* looked at 2500 autopsies conducted between 1979 and 1994. Researchers found that about 65% of men and 55% of women ages 65 and older had blockages extensive enough to be called severe coronary artery disease. They didn't necessarily die from the blockages, mind you. They just happened to have them. The older you are, the more likely you are to have blockages. By age 80, for example, 75% of people have significant blockages. By age 90, the number rises to 90%.

If you looked at the numbers alone, you would think that we're all headed for imminent heart attacks, and that older adults in their 80s and 90s would barely get enough blood to keep their hearts pumping. And yet, the vast majority of 90-year-olds have *no* symptoms of cardiac disease. Does that stop cardiologists from hauling out their Roto-Rooter tools? Of course not. If, for whatever reason, you get a complete heart work-up that includes an angiogram, you will almost certainly show signs of significant narrowing in your arteries. You might be perfectly healthy. You might not have any symptoms. But merely finding the problem almost guarantees that someone, sooner or later, will want to fix it.

Will fixing it make you better? Well, that depends on what you mean by "better." Yes, your heart will receive more blood than it did before. For surgeons who view every blockage as a problem, I suppose that's something. The more important question is whether surgery or other procedures will allow you live longer or feel healthier. The answer, in many cases, is no. If you can think of a better definition for "unnecessary surgery," let me know.

UNNECESSARY SURGERY?

Obviously, a blocked blood vessel that has caused a heart attack has to be opened. Surgery or other invasive procedures are also necessary for those with severe symptoms, or when medical management—aggressive changes in lifestyle habits along with the use of medications—hasn't worked. Opening the blood vessels surgically will virtually eliminate symptoms. But with a few exceptions, which I'll discuss below, doing surgery when there aren't clear-cut symptoms is a questionable practice, at best.

If diagnostic tests show that you have a significant degree of coronary artery disease, whether or not you have symptoms, you'll probably be advised to have one of two procedures: angioplasty (the full name is percutaneous transluminal coronary angioplasty), or bypass surgery (coronary artery bypass grafting). Together, more than a million and a half of these procedures are performed annually in the United States.

Angioplasty and Bypass Surgery

Angioplasty involves threading a narrow, sterile tube, with a tiny balloon at the tip, through a large blood vessel in the arm and leg. It snakes all the way up into the narrowed coronary artery, where the balloon is inflated. Pressure from the balloon mashes the thick layer of plaque tightly against the artery wall, just as squeezing a piece of bread makes it flatter. The inner diameter of the blood vessel gets larger, allowing more blood to pass through. In most cases, the surgeon will also insert a wire cage called a stent. It acts like scaffolding to keep the artery open.

Bypass surgery is a much more extensive procedure. The damaged sections of arteries are removed, then bypassed with healthy sections of blood vessels harvested from another part of the body—usually a vein from the leg, or from the internal mammary artery, an inessential blood vessel that carries blood to the breast. Bypass surgery requires stopping the heart temporarily and using a machine to route blood through the body during the procedure.

These procedures represent both the best and the worst of American medicine. Unless you've watched a surgeon at work, or seen the elaborate choreography that takes place in state-of-the-art operating rooms, it's hard to imagine the technical virtuosity that makes these procedures possible. People who have undergone angioplasty or bypass surgery almost revere their surgeons and cardiologists, and I can understand why. Yet we sometimes forget that technical ability isn't always the same thing as medical wisdom. Just because we *can* do these procedures doesn't mean we always should. They have become so routine that we tend to forget how serious they really are. Each procedure has a high risk of complications. The risks increase dramatically in older patients—the ones who are most likely to have the procedures done.

Weighing the Risks

More than 70% of bypass procedures are done on people 65 years and older. Patients are usually told that there's a 1 to 2% risk that they'll die during the surgery. That's hardly a walk in the park, but it doesn't sound so bad, either. Unfortunately, it's not the whole story. I have yet to meet a cardiac surgeon who quotes patients the death rates supported by Medicare statistics. The mortality rate of bypass surgery in those 65 to 69 years is 4.3%. In those 80 years and older, it's 10%. Within a year after having the surgery, the death rate is 8% in those 65 to 69, and 20% in those 80 and older.

Here are some of the other complications of bypass surgery:

• The risk of significant heart-rate irregularities following surgery approaches 50%.
• The risk of a having new heart attack is 6%.
• The risk of suffering a major stroke is about 2%.

- The risk of developing a serious, potentially life-threatening post-operative infection is close to 40%.
- There may be a higher than 40% risk of experiencing serious, irreversible cognitive declines, a consequence of reduced brain circulation and low body temperature during the procedure.
- The brain trauma caused by bypass surgery is likely to aggravate symptoms of Alzheimer's, a disease that's present in more than 50% of those over age 85.

You can see why I sometimes worry when my patients tell me that their cardiologists have advised them to have bypass surgery. I don't feel a whole lot better about angioplasty. It's not as invasive as surgery, but the risks are still high. The risk of a heart attack after angioplasty is about 6%. A study that looked at 633 patients, published in the *Journal of the American College of Cardiology,* found that 9% died in the hospital after angioplasty. The procedure also has a significant risk of causing uncontrolled bleeding or blood vessel damage. This occurs in about 3 to 5% of patients—and when it does, emergency bypass surgery may be the only option.

Even surgeons who acknowledge the published statistics tend to claim that the high potential risks don't reflect *their* risks. I don't think I've ever met a surgeon who rates his or her skills as average. Surgeons will tell patients that they have so much experience, and have done so many of the procedures, that the generally accepted risk figures don't apply to them. Obviously, an experienced surgeon who performs a lot of procedures gets very good at what he or she does. This does go a long way toward reducing complications. But the risks are still high, especially among older adults. Any surgeon who says otherwise isn't telling the whole truth.

There will be times when patients are obvious candidates for one of these procedures. Given the high risk of complications, they should be performed only when absolutely necessary—to open a recently blocked blood vessel that's resulted in a heart attack, for example. Immediately opening a blocked vessel can prevent permanent damage to the heart muscle. The procedures should also be done when patients are experiencing significant symptoms that can't be controlled in any other way, or when doctors conclude that the procedures will clearly prolong their lives.

If your cardiologist advises you to undergo one of these procedures, review the criteria above. Ask the cardiologist or surgeon if the procedure will achieve one or more of these goals. If the answer isn't a clear-cut yes, get a second opinion—fast. Your doctor may be pushing you toward a procedure you don't really need.

THE TRUTH ABOUT TREADMILL TESTS

If you're 40 years or older, you may have been advised by your primary care physician to start getting an annual treadmill stress test, a relatively low-cost way to detect coronary artery disease. During the test, you'll walk on a treadmill that gradually increases the level of exertion. Your heart will be monitored with an EKG. The goal of the test is to detect symptoms or heart-beat electrical changes that occur when the heart is starved for blood during exercise.

The rationale that's given for the test is that more than 50% of sudden heart attacks are the first "symptom" of coronary artery disease. These first heart attacks are often deadly, so it would seem to make sense to detect coronary artery disease at the earliest possible stage.

Treadmill stress tests may detect coronary artery disease, but they *don't* always predict heart attacks. Many individuals with normal stress test results suddenly get heart attacks due to blockages in apparently unaffected blood vessels. The tests can pick up obvious blood vessel abnormalities, but they don't seem to have much impact in real life.

The more critical issue, to my way of thinking, is that stress tests that show abnormal results tend to lead to unnecessary angioplasty or bypass operations. The man I described earlier is a perfect example. He had no symptoms whatsoever, but the test showed potential trouble. Off to the operating room he went. He wasn't sick before the surgery, but he was sure sick afterward. This is a tragedy—and an outrage.

Cardiologists often argue that treadmill stress tests are valuable because they alert patients to potential problems—that they serve as a valuable wake-up call. I suppose this is valid, up to a point. A patient who is prepared to make all of the necessary changes that have been shown to prevent coronary artery disease—quitting smoking, exercising, eating nutritious foods, lowering cholesterol, and so on—might benefit from knowing there's a potential problem. Of course, patients who are willing to make all of these changes don't need stress tests. Does it really help to raise the red flag when we all know what needs to be done? As for patients who won't make the necessary lifestyle changes, well, the tests might not do them much good, either.

There is one form of coronary artery disease that is very serious and is helped substantially by surgery. This is called isolated left main disease, in which only the left main coronary artery is affected. Many have suggested that a reason for a screening treadmill stress test is to identify this form of coronary artery disease, which if present should be corrected by surgery or angioplasty that will reduce the risk of heart attack and prolong your life. Lifestyle changes won't help if you have left main disease. You're going to need angioplasty or bypass surgery to reduce the risk of heart attack and prolong your life. But I can't imagine advising everyone to have a stress test on the off chance that they might have left main disease. It only affects about 5% of patients with coronary artery disease, and 97% of these have obvious symptoms. Left main disease is so rare, and it announces itself so clearly, that routine screenings to detect it are entirely unnecessary.

This isn't just my opinion, by the way. Most professional medical groups, among them the U.S. Preventive Services Task Force, do not recommend routine stress tests. Even the American College of Cardiology advises against routine testing, except for those who are about to launch into vigorous exercise program or to identify heart disease in those for whom a heart attack could affect public safety, such as pilots. The American College of Sports Medicine and the American Heart Association do recommend stress testing, but only for men 45 years and older who are about to participate in vigorous exercise. I've tried to figure out why so many doctors perform routine stress tests on so many patients, but there doesn't always seem to be a good reason.

Here's the bottom line. If you've been sedentary for years and suddenly get it into your head to change your ways and start training for a marathon, by all means get a stress test. It's an excellent way to detect exercise-induced changes in the cardiovascular system that could indicate coronary artery disease. If you're a smoker or have other risk factors for coronary artery disease, the test might be your wake-up call—but from a strictly medical point of view, it's unlikely to do you much good. Changing your habits will.

Save Your Money on CTs

Incidentally, you may have read media reports about electron-beam CT scans, a relatively new technique that identifies calcification of arterial plaque, a good measure of the severity of coronary artery disease. If the test identifies narrowing of one or more blood vessels, it's usually followed by a treadmill stress test to determine how much the narrowing is affecting blood supply. The test is all the rage, and a lot of testing clinics advertise low-cost screenings directly to consumers. My advice: Save your money. The procedure is even less useful than stress tests at predicting heart attacks. Quite a few studies have looked at this. The overwhelming conclusion is that merely identifying narrowed arteries serves no purpose in those who are symptom-free.

DEALING WITH SYMPTOMS: THE BEST WAYS TO EVALUATE AND TREAT CORONARY ARTERY DISEASE

So far, I've mainly talked about the limitations of testing and treatment in those who aren't having symptoms. But what if you have coronary artery disease and you are having symptoms? Obviously, the types of symptoms you're having, and their severity, will determine whether or not you need bypass surgery or angioplasty, or whether less invasive approaches will give better results.

One of the most typical early symptoms of coronary artery disease is angina, a sharp or pressing chest pain that occurs when narrowed coronary arteries are starving the heart of blood and oxygen. Angina is usually felt in the middle of the chest, and it frequently radiates into the neck and down the left arm. Many other conditions, including simple muscle strain, can cause chest pain that's easily confused with angina. What distinguishes angina is that it's usually brought on by exertion (or emotional stress). It never lasts longer than 30 minutes, and it quickly gets better when you rest. Some people, especially women and the elderly, are more likely to have what's called atypical angina. Rather than having chest pain, they may notice discomfort in the abdomen or back, or only in the arm or neck.

An irregular heartbeat is another symptom of coronary artery disease. People frequently get short of breath, especially during exertion, and they may have nausea or vomiting.

If you have recently developed any of these symptoms, see your physician immediately. It's not uncommon for angina and other symptoms to persist for years without causing additional problems, but neither is it uncommon for these symptoms to precede a heart attack. Your doctor will probably recommend that you have either a treadmill or thallium stress test, and perhaps an echocardiogram. If tests indicate that you do indeed have coronary artery disease, your doctor will likely schedule you for an angiogram. Let's take a look at these tests.

The Thallium/Treadmill Stress Test. The advantage of the thallium test is that it measures actual blood flow to the heart. You'll exercise on a treadmill while your heart is monitored. When you reach the point of fatigue, thallium, a radioactive substance that's taken up by the heart, is injected. A few minutes later, you'll lie down on an x-ray machine. The x-ray will reveal how much thallium reached the heart, which in turn indicates whether your blood supply is normal or not.

The Echocardiogram. In addition, an echocardiogram may be needed to evaluate your heart's ability to contract. The test measures the ejection fraction—the amount of blood that's pumped out with each beat. If the ejection fraction is less than 30%, you have a very high risk of dying from coronary artery disease, and you're more likely to need aggressive treatments.

The Angiogram. This test determines which blood vessels are blocked, and how severely. If you're lucky, the blockage may be in one of the minor, almost inconsequential, blood vessels. More often, the angiogram will reveal that three or more of the coronary arteries are blocked.

Left Main Disease

Less often, an angiogram will show blockage only in the left main coronary artery. This is the isolated left main disease I discussed earlier. Left main disease is serious business. If it's diagnosed during an angiogram, your cardiologist probably won't let you leave the hospital. You're going to need immediate surgery to undo the blockage. Surgery in this case can save your life. The five-year survival rate in those with left main disease is about 90% when they have surgery. Without surgery, the five-year survival rate is only about 60%. Fortunately, left main disease is fairly rare.

Triple Vessel Disease and Bypass Surgery

The common scenario in symptomatic patients is triple vessel disease. I wish I could say conclusively that surgery is or isn't the best option for triple vessel disease, but it's an incredibly complicated issue. God knows that it's scary to learn that virtually all of your coronary arteries are blocked. I can understand why so many patients, with the encouragement of their doctors, rush into surgery. Angioplasty, the less invasive procedure, is certainly an option, but the blockage comes back in one to two years in more than 50% of cases. Bypass surgery tends to give better results, but the question remains: Do you really need it?

Here are some guidelines that may be useful. These mainly apply to people between the ages of 50 and 70.

• Bypass surgery is the treatment of choice if you have triple vessel disease and you've also been diagnosed with diabetes. Angioplasty isn't an option in this case because it has a poorer success rate.

• You'll need bypass surgery if you have triple vessel disease that's accompanied by a low ejection fraction. If the heart muscle is so damaged that the ejection fraction—the amount of blood it can pump—is below 30%, opening the blood vessels with angioplasty won't help because the heart still won't be able to pump enough blood.

• If you have triple vessel disease, but the heart is functioning normally and you don't have diabetes, you might need surgery only if—out of stubbornness or an instinct toward self-destruction—you refuse to take medications or make the necessary lifestyle changes, such as lowering cholesterol, exercising, or quitting smoking.

This last point is worth repeating. Even if you have triple vessel disease that's causing symptoms, there's no good evidence that angioplasty or bypass surgery will necessarily provide any greater benefits than medical treatments or changing unhealthy habits. Besides, even if you opt for surgery, there's a good chance the blockages will come back, particularly if you don't take very good care of yourself. Thus, a man who has the surgery in his 50s may need a second procedure in 10 years. Second procedures are far more likely to cause death and lead to serious complications than first procedures. Delaying the time to first or second procedures is very much to your advantage.

NOT ALL PROCEDURES ARE EFFECTIVE

The groundbreaking work of Dr. Dean Ornish has clearly shown that people with coronary artery disease who exercise regularly, eat nutritiously, lower their cholesterol, and practice stress-reduction techniques do just as well as those who have angioplasty or bypass surgery. Indeed, the rigorous lifestyle changes Dr. Ornish recommends have been shown to reverse buildups of arterial plaque. People with angina who follow his program, for example, have seen reductions in symptoms of 91%. Those who don't make lifestyle changes, by contrast, typically have a doubling of angina episodes.

Put aside the lifestyle issues for a moment. Even in patients who go about their merry, self-destructive ways, the evidence that surgery prolongs life in those with coronary artery disease is less than compelling. In the best surgical hands, and in patients who have been carefully selected, bypass surgery only prolongs life by an average of four months during the five years after the procedure. In the longer term, over periods of 10 to 20 years, surgery is no more effective than medical management.

A recent study that followed patients for 22 years found that surgery did not improve survival or reduce the risk of heart attack in low-risk patients—those without diabetes who had normal ejection fractions. Even in high-risk patients, surgery only appears to improve survival in the first 10 years. Over longer periods, it doesn't add much to the equation. This is an important distinction because many people who have bypass surgery are treated at a relatively early age. They have a good number of years ahead of them, and you have to wonder why their doctors talk them into surgery when long-term medical management appears to work just as well. Besides, there's a 30% chance that people in their 50s, 60, or 70s who have bypass surgery will need a second procedure within 10 years. The mortality for second surgeries, even in those under age 70, is 10%. I don't know about you, but those odds don't give me a lot of confidence.

Cardiologists are well aware of the risks of surgery, even if they seem to underestimate them on occasion. More and more patients these days are being advised to have angioplasty. It's obviously less traumatic than surgery, and if I had to choose one or the other for low-risk patients with coronary artery disease, I'd certainly lean toward angioplasty. But the choice is between a rock and a hard place. Half or more of patients who undergo angioplasty have a recurrence of artery narrowing within a year. So they go through the procedure again—and believe me, it's no small thing. It might be less of an ordeal than surgery, but it's still a risky, invasive procedure. And remember, many of the patients who undergo the procedure have no, or only mild, symptoms.

An editorial in the *American Journal of Cardiology*, entitled "Need for a Moratorium on Percutaneous Transluminal Coronary Angioplasty in Stable Coronary Artery Disease," noted that there is *no* evidence that angioplasty offers any benefit over medical management. It beats me how any rational person could recommend invasive, potentially life-threatening procedures when patients could do just as well by improving health habits and, when necessary, taking relatively low-risk prescription drugs.

DEVASTATING FOR THE ELDERLY

I think that one of the biggest mistakes in modern medicine is the tendency of cardiologists and surgeons to be excessively aggressive in treating the elderly, those in their 70s and 80s, for coronary artery disease. As the elderly population increases, there's been an astronomical increase in the use of angioplasty and bypass surgery. More than 60% of these procedures are done in adults 65 years and older. The procedure rate almost doubled between 1987 and 1990, and then tripled in the next decade. For the life of me, I can't find anything in the medical literature that could possibly justify this staggering increase.

Angioplasty or surgery should never be performed on older adults if the goal is to prolong life or prevent another heart attack. No good research has shown that the procedures will achieve either one of these goals. The only reason to do these procedures in older patients is to restore blood flow following a heart attack, or when medical management to treat coronary artery disease has failed—when patients continue to have symptoms even when they make the necessary lifestyle changes and take drugs such as beta-blockers, calcium channel blockers, ACE inhibitors, or nitroglycerin. But for patients without symptoms? No, no, no!

Perhaps the most frustrating part of my practice is trying to convince patients with triple vessel disease that they don't need urgent surgery, no matter what their cardiologists might tell them. One of my patients, an 80-year-old man, showed evidence of inadequate coronary blood flow during an annual treadmill stress test. A follow-up angiogram confirmed that he had narrowed coronary arteries, and his cardiologist told him that he needed bypass surgery to reduce the risk of a heart attack. Keep in mind that this man had no symptoms at all. He didn't have diabetes and his heart function was good. I almost begged him not to have the surgery, but he said he wouldn't rest easy until the "problem" was fixed—never mind that he'd almost certainly had narrowed arteries for many, many years and was doing just fine. I told him that blockages occur slowly—so slowly, in fact, that had he had the angiogram 15 years ago, it probably would have shown about the same results. But I couldn't convince him. He went ahead and had the surgery. He did well initially, then died five days later when one of the repaired blood vessels ruptured.

I don't fault the surgeon's expertise. I know his work, and he's one of the best in the business. But I do fault a health system that's intent on identifying, and fixing, anatomical abnormalities, whether or not these abnormalities have any practical impact on peoples' lives. In this case, the man clearly should have been managed with medical and lifestyle measures. He wasn't sick. He wasn't having symptoms. All he had was evidence of potential problems—problems that in all likelihood could have been avoided *without* high-risk interventions. If nothing else, his doctor should have initially advised watchful waiting—keeping an eye on the man to see how he did over a few months or years. Surgery could always be done later if his condition worsened. But instead, surgery was the first, not the last choice, and the poor man paid the price. So if you or someone in your family has coronary artery disease, please, don't be in a hurry to call in the surgeons.

Change Your Lifestyle First

I've explained some of the circumstances when angioplasty or bypass surgery are clearly indicated—when you're having symptoms, or when a blockage has resulted in a heart attack. If these circumstances don't apply to you, and they don't for a majority of people, you probably don't need surgery right away. What you do need, urgently, is to make some lifestyle changes. These include:

Keep a low-fat diet. Studies have shown conclusively that reducing fat intake to less than 30% of total calories is among the best ways to prevent fatty deposits from accumulating in the coronary arteries. Dean Ornish recommends a strict vegetarian diet, but I think this is excessive for most people. You'll do fine if you keep dietary fat at reasonable levels.

Stop smoking. It's an absolute must. Smoking damages artery linings and dramatically increases arterial narrowing. It also increases the risk of irregular heartbeats called arrhythmias. If you quit smoking, your risk of having a heart attack will decline to the levels of life-long nonsmokers within a few years.

Exercise for 30 minutes at least three days a week. More is better.

Manage daily stress. Exercise, do meditation, take up yoga—whatever works for you. The evidence is very clear that stress dramatically increases the risk of heart disease.

Aggressively lower your cholesterol. Some people can do it by reducing the amount of saturated fat in their diets. Others may need statins or other cholesterol-lowering drugs. Elevated cholesterol is among the main risk factors for coronary artery disease.

Take half an aspirin—or one baby aspirin—daily. Aspirin reduces the clotting action of cell-like structures in blood called platelets. Most heart attacks occur when clots in the arteries prevent blood from reaching the heart.

Be conscientious about controlling your blood pressure. Even mildly elevated blood pressure damages blood vessels and increases the risk of heart attack. You want to keep your systolic pressure (the first number) below 135; the diastolic pressure should be lower than 90.

Every day, take 1000 micrograms of vitamin B12 and 400 micrograms of folic acid. These nutrients lower levels of homocysteine, an amino acid that's been linked to heart disease.

Conservative treatments are surprisingly effective. The drugs used to treat coronary artery disease can reduce or even eliminate symptoms. Lifestyle changes can ease symptoms, help you feel better, and possibly reverse some of the underlying problems. Dean Ornish's research suggests that more than 80% of patients with coronary artery disease will improve significantly when they combine medical management with lifestyle changes.

There are limits to medical management, of course. If you're one of the unlucky ones, you may need angioplasty or bypass surgery. There's nothing wrong with either of these procedures—they can, in fact, dramatically improve your quality of life by eliminating or reducing symptoms that weren't helped by conservative measures. But think of them, always, as last resorts. Don't risk your health by correcting problems that may not need to be fixed.

If You've Already Had a Heart Attack

While I strongly advise conservative therapy for most patients, an exception must be made for those who have had heart attacks. Most heart attack patients are immediately given thrombolytic therapy—drugs such as streptokinase or tissue plasminogen activator, which dissolve clots and restore blood flow to the heart. When the drugs are given early enough, they can prevent damage to the heart muscle. After thrombolytic therapy, most patients are given an angiogram to identify blood vessels blockages that allowed clots to form in the first place. After this, they usually need angioplasty to open the blockages and improve circulation to the heart.

A recent study in the *Journal of the American Medical Association* reported that heart attack patients who underwent angioplasty lived longer and were less likely to suffer heart damage than those who got thrombolytic therapy alone. It seems likely that angioplasty will soon be the standard treatment for patients who have had a sudden heart attack, also called acute myocardial infarction. It may be especially beneficial for elderly heart attack patients, for whom the risks of thrombolytic therapy, such as uncontrolled bleeding, are very high. Also, older patients have relatively little cardiac "reserve." They simply can't afford to lose additional heart function following a heart attack, and angioplasty minimizes this risk.

While I favor conservative measures for older adults with asymptomatic coronary artery disease, and for those whose symptoms can be managed with drugs or lifestyle changes, I think we should be much more aggressive in dealing with heart attacks. Doctors are often reluctant to trot out angioplasty or the other big guns for patients who are old and sick. It's true that the risks of surgical complications are higher in older adults, but the benefits are sufficiently dramatic to justify going ahead.

BE TRUE TO YOUR HEART

Coronary artery disease is in some ways a very straightforward problem. Arteries are narrowed or blocked with fatty deposits. The heart doesn't get enough blood, which may—or may not—cause symptoms, such as chest pain, breathlessness, and fatigue. Coronary artery disease greatly increases your risk of a heart attack. You have to deal with it. Based on the best available research, here's what you need to do.

Do everything you can to prevent coronary artery disease. Most cases are linked to lifestyle. If you take this approach seriously—by getting plenty of exercise, lowering cholesterol, not smoking, and so on—you can almost guarantee you won't get it.

Unless your doctor specifically tells you otherwise, don't bother with routine treadmill stress tests or CT scans to detect coronary artery disease. The only reason to get screened, in the absence of symptoms, is if you're about to embark on a vigorous exercise program.

If you have stable coronary artery disease—that is, your blood vessels show signs of narrowing, but you aren't having symptoms, or the symptoms you do have aren't getting worse—don't rush into angioplasty or bypass surgery. Push your doctor hard for answers. If he or she can't make a convincing case that the procedures will make you feel better, lengthen your life, or prevent a heart attack, don't have them.

Angioplasty and bypass surgery are major procedures with a significant risk of complications—complications that can be more dangerous than the disease itself. The potential effects on long-term memory are of particular concern, especially in those 70 years and older.

Do consider bypass surgery if your coronary artery disease is accompanied by diabetes, or if your heart's ability to pump blood is significantly reduced. These are two cases in which surgery has clearly been shown to be beneficial.

If you've had a heart attack, encourage your doctors to treat it aggressively, no matter how old you are. Angioplasty to open clogged vessels has clearly been shown to protect the heart better than drug therapy alone.

CHAPTER THREE

*"I bought some ginkgo biloba to help with my memory, but I
keep forgetting to take it!"*   —*Marilyn, age 64*

WHEN NATURAL
ISN'T BETTER

S urveys show that the majority of Americans turn to alternative
therapies—everything from herbal remedies and nutritional
extracts to superhigh doses of vitamins or minerals—on occasion, and some use them all the time. Between 1990 and 1997, for example, there was a 380% increase in the use of herbal remedies, and a 130%
increase in the use of high-dose vitamins.

The allure of alternative therapies seems to be the belief that these
approaches are somehow more natural—and hence beneficial—than
mainstream medicine. Nature is thought to be benevolent and wholesome. Natural approaches and products are perceived as safer than synthetic drugs, more in tune with the body than high-tech medical
approaches.

But this "natural is better" argument strikes me as a singularly poor
reason to choose one health approach over another. There's nothing
about nature that's especially benign. Think about malaria, anthrax, cancer. Or cyanide or strychnine, for that matter. Natural, yes. Wholesome

and benign, hardly! I can't imagine why anyone would deliberately turn their backs on approaches that have been proven to work in favor of treatments of questionable value—or that have been proven to have *no value*—merely because they're natural.

There is no compelling evidence that the majority of alternative remedies and techniques do what they're said to do. And yet, they do contain chemically active compounds that affect bodily functions just as much as any prescription drug. This means they aren't without risk. Personally, if I'm going to put a chemical in my body, I want to choose one that's been exhaustively studied. It might not be free of side effects, but at least someone has taken the time to study the risks as well as the benefits. With most alternative remedies, you're taking the word of manufacturers and the touts on late-night TV or on the Internet. I know which source of information I trust. But I suspect I may be in the minority.

THE ALTERNATIVE EXPLOSION

A Harvard study in 1997 found that 67% of Americans have used at least one form of alternative therapy, and it's likely that this number will rise in the years to come. Among the elderly, who presumably are more conservative than their younger peers, 30% said they used alternative remedies. The percentage jumped to 50% among baby boomers.

As more and more people show an interest in nontraditional treatments, there's a corresponding increase in practitioners. In 1997, for example, Americans made 629 million visits to practitioners of alternative therapy. That's substantially more than the number of visits to primary care physicians.

Some of my more conservative colleagues take a dark view of this state of affairs. They mutter that people who turn to alternative medicine are putting their lives on the line, at least in those cases when they neglect conventional treatments for cancer or other serious conditions. I have to say, this concern is a little bit of a stretch. There are charlatans out there who prey on cancer patients and others with life-threatening conditions. And some patients do turn their backs entirely on mainstream medicine. But a little perspective is in order. The majority of alternative therapies are aimed at relatively minor, if chronic, health problems, such as back pain, fatigue, indigestion, or headache—the same conditions, incidentally, that mainstream medicine has been the least helpful in treating. Given our dismal success rates for back pain, for example, it's certainly understandable that patients would seek other options.

Today I had lunch with a good friend who happens to be one of my patients. As always, she talked at length about her distrust of Western medicine in general and physicians (myself excepted, apparently) in particular. In the years I've known her, she's probably used, and sworn by, hundreds of alternative remedies. Her most recent discovery, I learned, is aloe gel for ulcers. She likes it a lot better than the prescription drugs I'd prescribed. The drugs didn't work very well, she explained, and the gel provided nearly instant relief.

I'm not familiar with any research that suggests that aloe gel works for gastrointestinal complaints. I don't have a clue what active compounds it contains. Still, I'm never one to argue with success. If she thinks it works, and it doesn't cause side effects, why not?

But I can't help but wonder what has led her—along with so many of my patients—to put their trust in remedies that probably have never been tested, are unregulated by the FDA or other health agencies, and have no readily identifiable mechanisms that suggest they'd be effective. This patient, along with millions of like-minded Americans, doesn't hesitate to take handfuls of these products every day. One time, out of curiosity, I asked her to describe everything she was currently taking. The list below is by no means complete, but it does give a sense of her dedication.

- Vitamin E for its antioxidant properties
- Alpha-lipoic acid for carbohydrate metabolism and fat deactivation
- DHEA to prevent wrinkles and improve mood and memory
- Coenzyme Q-10 for heart and gum health
- Grape seed extract for everything from heart and lung health to cancer prevention
- Fish oil for arthritis and to lower cholesterol
- Flax seed oil to lower cholesterol, increase energy and vitality, and strengthen the nails
- Red yeast rice to lower cholesterol
- Enzymes for improved digestion
- Evening primrose oil for the heart and to control inflammation
- Hawthorne for the heart
- Estriol, a plant estrogen, for hormone replacement
- Turmeric root for pain
- Chelation therapy to detoxify the body and remove fat from the arteries

I confess, my mouth fell open as she recited her alternative A-list. I try to be open-minded, but most of these "remedies" are so outlandish, and so unlikely to have any benefits, that I had to ask her what the hell she thought she was doing. She wasn't abashed by my question at all. As a Christian, she explained, she'd rather use medicines from nature because they come from God. Doesn't it make more sense, she asked, to go right to the source and bypass the "middle man"?

If I've made her sound a little kooky, it's only because I haven't told the whole story. As with many of my patients who take the alternative approach, she has hardly given up conventional care. She takes prescription drugs to lower cholesterol and blood pressure. She comes in for checkups regularly, and for the most part she does all the things—regular exercise, a reasonable diet, and so on—that she needs to be healthy. She depends on the best of modern medicine, and then she makes up her own mind about therapies that are outside the medical mainstream. Is she—and the many others like her—wasting their money? Or do they know a few things that medical professionals don't?

Seeking Solutions Elsewhere

People who utilize the alternative approach aren't delusional. Many of them recognize the weaknesses, or at least the uncertain outcomes, of alternative approaches. Yet they use them anyway. Is it because terms like "holistic" and "natural" have such an irresistible pull? Or is because I and my colleagues are somehow pushing them away from everything we represent?

Anyone who's old enough to have witnessed the changes in our health care system over the last few decades can't help but be dismayed. We've all encountered the worst of HMOs. The callous indifference to suffering, the inability to see the doctors of our choice, the seemingly irrational denial of what should be obvious benefits are hardly the qualities that bind us to mainstream medicine. We all sympathize when our doctors seem to be overworked and overwhelmed. It's a lot harder to feel compassion when their arrogance precedes them like a black cloud. They buzz in and out of the examining room. Maybe they introduce themselves, maybe they don't. They ask questions without really listening to the answers.

I recently learned that the average amount of time patients spend with doctors is about six minutes. Six minutes! That's barely enough time to deal with whatever it is that brought you in the door, let alone getting a good sense of your overall health or concerns. Before a word has come out of your mouth, it seems, a prescription has been written. Not a mention of health promotion or prevention. No questions about your family, your job, your worries. Just an automaton in a white coat. No wonder so many people are looking elsewhere for solutions.

BIG CLAIMS, DOUBTFUL BENEFITS

My objection to most alternative approaches isn't that they're new (many have been used for thousands of years), or that I didn't learn about them in medical school. The problem is that most of the "natural" treatments used by my patients have never been tested. We don't know who they'll help and who they'll hurt. We don't know for sure what side effects they'll cause. We don't know how they compare to other, possibly better, treatments. How can I recommend alternative remedies when there's hardly a shred of evidence that they work?

I sincerely believe that there is a role for nature's medicines in treating illness. I, too, am jaded by the current medical system's emphasis on profits and cost containment. But the widespread belief that herbs, supplements, and other natural products are better and less harmful than drugs is seriously flawed.

St. John's Wort for Depression?

Here's an example. I suspect that nearly half of my patients take St. John's wort. An herb commonly used in supplement form, St. John's wort has been recommended for the treatment of depression. I understand the appeal. Prescription antidepressants are rife with side effects, including low energy, malaise, and sexual dysfunction. St. John's wort is less likely to cause serious side effects, and many people are convinced that it works. Does it really?

Let me start by saying that all depression isn't the same. There is some scientific data that suggests that St. John's wort can help alleviate symptoms of mild to moderate depression. But major depression is a different creature, one that requires entirely different approaches. Unfortunately, alternative practitioners and supplement manufacturers rarely make this important distinction. Major depression—which is defined by the National Institutes of Mental Health as experiencing depression or a lack of interest in normal activities for most of the day, every day for about two weeks, and also having symptoms such as weight gain, sleep disturbances, or thoughts of suicide—is a serious illness. For alternative practitioners to recommend an herbal treatment with thin research behind it is careless in the extreme.

Researchers recently conducted a large, double-blind clinical study that compared St. John's wort to placebo for the treatment of moderate to severe depression. The report, which appeared in the *Journal of the American Medical Association*, found that people taking St. John's wort did no better than those taking placebo. To put it another way, taking this herb for serious depression is no more effective than drinking a glass of water.

Not everyone who takes St. John's wort is seriously depressed, of course. Many of my patients take it when they're dealing with temporary upsets in their lives, or because they're feeling tired and run down. One of my patients, for example, started taking St. John's wort after her son nearly died from an alcohol binge. As she described it to me, her mood was much improved two to three days after taking the supplements. Well, guess what? St. John's wort doesn't work that way. Even the studies that suggest it's effective for mild depression have shown that it takes at least two weeks to work. My patient credited the herb with helping her feel better, but the real credit goes to the placebo effect—the power of the mind to influence the body. She thought the supplements would work, and so they did. A sugar pill would have done the same thing.

I'm all for trying new things. If St. John's wort were truly harmless, I'd have no objection to it. But side effects, such as anxiety, agitation, and confusion, aren't uncommon. The herb increases the risk of internal bleeding when it's combined with Coumadin, a blood-thinning drug. It appears to interact with some contraceptives and with medications used to treat HIV. It may also cause serious side effects when it's combined with mainstream antidepressants.

Apart from the herb's questionable safety profile and limited benefits, I worry that people with serious depression will depend on it or other alternative treatments when what they desperately need is professional help. Major depression is a life-threatening condition. Self-treatment with an herbal product—with or without the supervision of an alternative practitioner—is a very dangerous path.

Kava for Anxiety?

Another popular herb these days is kava, commonly used to treat anxiety. Some studies from Europe suggest that it may be helpful, and the National Center for Complementary and Alternative Medicine, a part of the National Institutes of Health, recently launched a large-scale, multicenter study to examine its potential benefits. Soon after the study began, however, reports began to emerge linking kava with serious liver damage. The researchers determined that the risks were so great that the study has been put on hold for the time being.

Kava isn't alone in causing side effects, of course. The same could be said of many mainstream prescription and over-the-counter drugs. It may turn out that the benefits of kava, like its pharmaceutical counterparts, will outweigh the potential risks. But it's important to remember that "natural" drugs are still drugs. The use of these products is far from risk-free. It doesn't matter whether you brew them in a tea or pop them in capsule form. As for kava, my advice is simple: Don't go near it.

Ginseng for Everything?

Finally, I'd like to touch on ginseng, an herbal therapy that has been recommended for just about every condition imaginable, from low energy to diabetes. Frankly, I think ginseng represents alternative therapy at its worst. Any time a product is touted as a cure-all, you can bet that it's unlikely to work for much of anything. I'm not aware of any good studies on ginseng that have shown measurable benefits.

PREYING ON THE MOST VULNERABLE

Infomercials fill the airways on many cable channels, as well as on the local networks in the late evening and early morning hours. The ones selling health products always intrigue me, and I watch them often. They feature nice-looking doctors, a slew of grateful "patients," and promises of everything but eternal life. For entertainment value—or for help with the occasional bout of insomnia—the programs aren't bad. I find it difficult to believe that anyone takes the promises seriously, but apparently millions do.

Most of the products sold on TV and the Internet are relatively innocuous. Take the so-called stress formulas. There's not a hint of evidence that any combination of herbs, vitamins, or minerals will help you cope with stress any better than you did before. The products won't improve your energy, your sex life, or physical performance. They won't "detoxify" your body, whatever that means. They're pure snake oil. Even so, these ads don't bother me too much because they're targeting people with relatively minor problems. They might be rip-offs, but they're unlikely to do any harm.

Unfortunately, this isn't always the case. A great many alternative approaches and remedies give false hope to people with serious, potentially life-threatening conditions. And in more than a few cases, the products themselves may be dangerous.

Diet products are a prime example. The quacks, playing on peoples' insecurity about their weight, promote "fat-busting" pills, powders, and potions—all-natural products that they claim will stimulate the metabolism and cause fat to melt away like hot butter.

Forget for a moment that none of these claims has any scientific basis in fact. (Many products contain nothing more than amino acids, vitamins, and minerals. Think of them as very expensive multivitamins.) The main issue, to me, is that some of the ingredients may be dangerous. This is especially true of ephedra, a staple of Traditional Chinese Medicine. Ephedra contains a chemical compound called ephedrine, which is known to cause cardiac irregularities, especially in those with high blood pressure. A suit was recently filed in New York state by the husband of a woman who died suddenly while exercising on a treadmill, and who had been taking ephedra as an appetite suppressant.

Lessons from Laetrile

Far worse than the promotion of natural diet products is the vast, unregulated market that preys on the desperation of those with cancer, AIDS, or other life-threatening illnesses. Studies suggest that the underground market for untested, unproven, and possibly unsafe cancer remedies is vast. More than 60% of cancer patients get some of their information from this alternative realm, and all too many choose these routes of treatment at the expense of conventional care. The most vulnerable entrust their lives—and turn over their bank accounts—to nutritional or alternative cancer clinics in the United States and abroad. The results are nothing short of horrifying.

The laetrile fiasco is a prime example. The active ingredient in laetrile is amygdaline, a compound that contains high concentrations of cyanide and was reputed to shrink tumors. Early research by the National Cancer Institute and others found no evidence that it had this effect, and the side effects, mainly those of cyanide poisoning, included liver damage, low blood pressure, coma, and even death. Yet it was given to thousands of desperate cancer patients before being banned in the United States and most other countries about fifteen years ago.

Even though laetrile has been roundly discredited, its supposed benefits still circulate widely in the alternative medicine community. You would think that the clear evidence that it doesn't work would bury it for good. Not so. As recently as 2001, the *Los Angeles Times* published a letter to the editor from G. Edward Griffin, the founder of a group called Cancer Cure Foundation, who argues that the negative laetrile findings were due to poor or fraudulent research. Regrettably, that's a common theme among the hard-core adherents of alternative approaches. They believe mainstream science is corrupt, incompetent, or beholden to the interests of large drug manufacturers. Negative findings, in this view, don't mean a drug or treatment isn't effective, only that researchers are too blinded by vested interests to give impartial judgments.

Laetrile is probably the most publicized of the alternative, and bogus, cancer treatments, but it's hardly the only one. One that's been cropping up lately is a "drug" called 714X, whose developer had to leave France for practicing medicine without a license. Others products include AMP, which is derived from mushrooms and is said to have eliminated cancer in 90% of experimental animals; chelation therapy with the chemicals DMSO and EDTA; and nutritional supplements that are said to enhance the ability of the immune system to destroy tumors or prevent their growth. There's not a shred of evidence that any of these approaches is effective. Oncologists roll their eyes when they hear about them. And yet, people keep using them. Amazing.

False Hope for Cancer Patients

Earlier this year, a *Primetime* special called "False Promises" followed reporter Chris Wallace and a breast cancer patient as they toured alternative cancer clinics in Tijuana, Mexico. Recommended treatments included coffee enemas, pressure chambers, electromagnetic therapy, and the use of a gizmo called an "ozonator." The costs of the treatments ranged from $15,000 to $30,000. The results, to put it mildly, were not promising.

One of the most remarkable arguments for alternative cancer therapy—and against mainstream medicine—comes from the Wellness Directory of Minnesota. It maintains that merely because a therapy is unproven doesn't mean it has been "disproven." I suppose this is true, as far as it goes. Researchers haven't investigated everything, and there's always the possibility that an unlikely hypothesis will turn out to be fact at some point. And let's face it, it's all but impossible to prove a negative. But scientists who spend their careers studying cancer or heart disease or HIV have a pretty good sense of what's possible and what's not. They don't need to waste time "disproving" ideas that can't possibly work.

Fraud, deception, false promises, and the prolongation of needless hope seem to be par for the course in the alternative-treatment community. It's tragic when patients, swayed by slick marketing campaigns, lose valuable time by pursuing unproven natural therapies, and reduce their chances of getting a good response or even a cure from conventional medical treatments. I have no objection, in principle, to the use of natural therapies. But there must be proof. There must be clear guidelines and objectives. Any cancer treatment, for example, should be expected to

- shrink or eliminate a tumor,
- result in a cure or disease-free remission,
- prolong life,
- relieve symptoms, or
- improve quality of life.

Any treatment that meets these goals, be it a conventional pharmaceutical or some yet-to-be-discovered plant compound, deserves attention. Testimonials aren't proof. The therapy must be tested against state-of-the-art treatments. It does not have to be a cure, but it must have some proven advantage that makes it possible to rationally recommend its use.

Government Watchdogs

The Federal Trade Commission (FTC) recently initiated a program called "Operation Cure.All," which is designed to combat Internet health fraud. According to Howard Beales, of the FTC's Bureau of Consumer Protection, the Internet has allowed "unscrupulous marketers to peddle products with unproven and false claims." Clearly, we all have to view the Internet, mass mailings, and other forms of advertising with a healthy degree of suspicion. This is especially true of those that promise miraculous cures for serious diseases.

As I mentioned before, I don't worry too much about products that do nothing worse than bilk consumers out of their disposable incomes.

I'd like to see the products be more closely regulated, but at least no one is seriously harmed. That's not always the case, however. Every day, it seems, the FDA or other health groups release warnings about various alternative remedies. For example:

• The FDA recently advised consumers about the dangers of a weight-loss product called Lipokinetix. It has been shown to cause liver damage and even liver failure. It contains ephedra, caffeine, yohimbine, diiodothyronine (a thyroid hormone), and sodium usniate. Who knows where these agents come from or what the rationale is for including them in the product? I don't.

• A product called Triax Metabolic Accelerator contains a potent thyroid hormone called triiodothyroacetic acid, which can cause anxiety, severe sweating, fast heart rate, and stroke.

• Dieter's Brews, teas that contain senna, aloe, buckthorn, and other plant-based laxatives, can cause diarrhea, dehydration, elevated heart rate, and other dangerous side effects.

The widespread frustration with our health care system, and the promise of safe, powerful alternatives that harness the forces of nature, make these and other "natural" therapies seem like very attractive options. More than 50% of cancer patients use one or more alternative therapies, and some may forsake traditional medicine altogether. This is tragic because not one of these approaches, to date, has proven more effective than conventional treatments.

THE PLUS SIDE OF NATURE'S MEDICINES

Unlike many of my colleagues, I do try to stay open-minded. Just because an herb or vitamin combination hasn't been proven to be effective doesn't mean it won't be at some time in the future. After all, many things that seem obvious to us today, like the existence of microscopic organisms or the importance of good hygiene, were viewed as rather on the fringes not that long ago. And to be perfectly honest, nature has given us an incredible wealth of treatments that we never would have dreamed up in the laboratory.

Many of the drugs we depend on, for example, are derived more or less directly from nature. Digitalis, a cornerstone in the treatment of heart failure, comes from the foxglove plant. Penicillin comes from a ground fungus. I could name hundreds of other examples. Today, these medicines are made entirely in the laboratory from synthetic materials, but they got their start in nature.

But this raises an interesting point. Would anyone, even someone who tilts toward the alternative end of the spectrum, insist on drinking foxglove tea rather than taking a precisely engineered pill? Nature provided the raw material, but it took modern technology and science to refine it into something that's effective, standardized, and predictable. Some doctors might dismiss "natural" remedies out of hand. Some patients dismiss mainstream treatments. But it seems to me that the best of all possible approaches is a fusion of the two.

Consider the drug paclitaxel (Taxol), which was first isolated from the Pacific yew tree by two scientists from the Research Triangle Institute in North Carolina. They found in animal studies that paclitaxel reduced the size of tumors. The success of subsequent clinical trials led Dr. Samuel Broder, the director of the National Cancer Institute, to call paclitaxel the most significant anticancer drug of the decade. For a long time, the Pacific yew was the only source of paclitaxel. It took the amount of paclitaxel in six 100-year-old trees to treat just one patient. If nature remained the only source of paclitaxel, the Pacific yew would rapidly disappear. Fortunately, talented chemists were able to create a semisynthetic form of the drug. It's virtually identical to the original, but it's made in a laboratory instead of stripped from the landscape—the perfect mix of nature and science.

So far, I've talked mainly about the risks of alternative remedies. I think it's worth pausing for a moment to consider why so many people take these products. One of the biggest reasons, I suspect, is the ability of the mind to influence the body and promote healing. Another term for this is the placebo effect. Study after study has shown that people who take "blank" pills, or placebos, often have a marked improvement in symptoms. In some cases, in fact, placebos have even caused tumors to temporarily shrink.

I'm not surprised that people who turn to alternative therapies often see benefits in the short run. The placebo effect clearly makes a difference. So do spiritual and emotional factors, which have been shown to improve health as well as longevity. People who turn to natural therapies often have a deep belief in the curative powers of nature. This belief by itself can make a difference in their long-term health.

Before most drugs are approved by the FDA, they have to be proved to be *more* effective than placebos. This type of research, the placebo-controlled clinical trial, is the gold standard in scientific research. In the last few years, more and more alternative therapies have been subjected to these tests. When carefully designed research studies clearly show that herbs or other natural products are superior to placebo, it's highly likely that these treatments will leave the realm of "alternative" and become routine parts of conventional treatments.

In the last few years, more and more conventional physicians have become convinced that some alternative therapies are, in fact, effective. I'd like to single these out for discussion because they're perfect examples of what happens when scientific research works the way it's supposed to. Let's suppose that scientists decide to investigate whether or not a particular therapy works. They design experiments that compare the therapy to placebo or other current treatments. If they discover benefits, the therapy enters the mainstream. If no benefits are revealed, the treatment is abandoned—or, too often, promoted on late-night TV or the Internet. Here are a couple of the clear winners.

Ginkgo

Herbalists have used it for centuries, and a preliminary research study published in *The Lancet* showed that it improved memory in patients with insufficient blood supply to the brain, a condition called vascular dementia. The researchers tested their hypothesis by giving patients memory tests before and after taking ginkgo, and the improvements were significant. I wouldn't have used gingko in the past, but based on this study, I now routinely recommend it to patients with vascular dementia.

I also recommend ginkgo to patients who get calf pain when they walk. This condition, called intermittent claudication, is caused by inadequate blood flow to the lower legs. Studies have shown that a chemical compound in ginkgo causes arteries in the legs to dilate and carry more blood.

The science is conclusive at this point that ginkgo is helpful for those with impaired blood flow. As often happens, however, the alternative medicine community has jumped on these findings, taken them out of context, and concluded, erroneously, that ginkgo improves memory and intellectual prowess in everyone. I recently heard that every member of a big-city symphony orchestra takes ginkgo before concerts to improve their performance!

Just to set the record straight: Even though ginkgo is a classic example of an herb that is active as a drug—one that relaxes blood vessels and improves blood flow—it's only effective when blood flow is impaired to begin with. There's absolutely no reason for healthy people to take it. It won't make your memory better than it was before, and it won't raise your IQ. It may cause side effects in some cases. Headaches are the main one. Bleeding problems, although not common, have been reported, and ginkgo may cause seizures if taken in high enough doses.

Saw Palmetto

It was probably the first herbal remedy I heard of, and the first one I used myself. A close friend of mine, a plastic surgeon, had suffered from prostate problems for years. He woke up six or seven times a night to go to the bathroom, and he always had trouble getting the flow going. Worse, he had what's known as "after-dribble," which resulted in little wet patches on his trousers after using the bathroom. Embarrassing, to say the least. His urologist recommend that he take saw palmetto, and apparently it worked very well. Being a man of a certain age myself, I read up on saw palmetto and decided it was worth a try. It didn't work miracles in my case, but there's enough evidence to suggest it works for prostate enlargement (called benign prostatic hypertrophy, or BPH) that I often recommend it to my male patients.

The studies I've seen suggest that saw palmetto works best for mild cases of BPH. In Europe, doctors consider it a front-line treatment. Side effects hardly ever occur, and the herb is a lot cheaper than the drugs commonly used to treat this problem. The only drawback that I can see is that saw palmetto may lower the concentration of prostate-specific antigen, a "marker" that's used to detect prostate cancer. In theory, this could make the cancer more difficult to detect, but I'm not sure that this is a significant issue.

Vitamin E

Vitamin E has long been a heavy hitter in the world of alternative nutrition. Vitamin E disciples have made all sorts of claims, from the reasonable to the outlandish. It's hardly a panacea, but it has been shown to have two important effects. It's an antioxidant that neutralizes highly toxic molecules that are naturally produced by cells in the process of metabolism. Under normal circumstances, these molecules, called superoxide and hydroxyl radicals, are neutralized by cell enzymes— enzymes that get less effective with age or illness. Vitamin E can take up the slack and prevent these molecules from damaging cells in the brain, blood vessels, and other parts of the body.

Vitamin E also reduces the ability of cell-like structures called platelets to clump together. This is important because these clumps, or clots, can restrict or stop blood flow and lead to heart attacks or strokes.

One large study found that the risk of second heart attacks was cut in half when patients took 800 international units of vitamin E daily. Other studies have shown that vitamin E can reduce the tendency of cholesterol to stick to artery walls. Finnish researchers who studied 27,000 men found that those who took vitamin E were 4% less likely to have a heart attack, and 8% less likely to have a fatal heart attack. Preliminary studies also suggest that vitamin E may slow the progression of Alzheimer's disease, probably because it reduces brain inflammation.

Based on this information, I recommend vitamin E to patients who either have had a heart attack or are at risk of getting one. I also recommend it to those with a family history or other risk factors for heart disease. While vitamin E may increase the risk of bleeding in some cases, this side effect is rare.

Vitamin B12

A deficiency of this nutrient—which can result in memory loss, balance problems, anemia, and other conditions—is very common after age 65. In fact, about 10% of older adults have vitamin B12 levels at the lower limit of the healthy range or below. In our clinic, we've found that about 15% of patients evaluated for memory disorders are low in vitamin B12.

The only dietary source of vitamin B12 is animal products, such as milk and meat. The only way the nutrient can be absorbed is when stomach acid levels are normal, and when a protein, called intrinsic factor, is produced by the stomach. But about 25% of people aged 70 and older don't produce enough stomach acid or intrinsic factor to ensure adequate B12 absorption.

It used to be thought that the only way to replace vitamin B12 was by injection. We now know that giving large oral doses—usually 500 to 1000 micrograms—works just as well. Even in large amounts, the nutrient causes no side effects, it's inexpensive, and it very clearly works. I now recommend vitamin B12 supplements to all of my patients who are 70 years and older. As a bonus, this vitamin also lowers levels of homocysteine, an amino acid that has been linked to heart disease.

• • •

These are the only alternative remedies that I routinely use in my practice. Why so few? Because they're the only ones, in my view, with enough scientific evidence behind them to warrant their use. They've been tested in carefully controlled clinical trials. The side effects are well documented. We know a lot about how they interact with other medications. In short, we know a great deal about them. I feel comfortable recommending them to my patients because I know they work.

In the cases of vitamins E and B12, it's worth noting that the beneficial effects stem from giving pharmacologic rather than nutritional doses. In other words, they work like drugs when they're given in large enough amounts. Vitamin E, gingko, and other alternative remedies may be natural substances, but they are drugs, no better and no worse. Along with their benefits comes the risk of side effects. Any drug, "natural" or otherwise, exerts effects on the body that range from mild to profound. But as long as we treat these remedies as drugs, and require the same burdens of proof, we're less likely to be blindsided by unsuspected risks or side effects.

There is clearly a place for alternative therapies in modern medicine. Some of these therapies are clearly beneficial as long as they're used appropriately. I'm grateful that the scientific community in general, and the National Institutes of Health in particular, are taking the use of alternative therapies seriously. The NIH has formed the National Center for Complementary and Alternative Medicine. Millions of dollars are now earmarked to study many different forms of alternative therapy. Carefully controlled clinical trials are now under way to evaluate the benefits and risks of these therapies. In the near future, I hope, we'll have hard facts to work with, facts that will undoubtedly document the benefits of some therapies, while discrediting others.

USING THEM WISELY

In my experience, the alternative remedies that are most likely to work are the ones that are targeted toward very specific goals, such as easing headache, diarrhea, or anxiety, for example. These are the ones that have been most rigorously studied. However, the more sweeping the claims, the more likely it is that the remedy will be ineffective. When you come across products that promise everything from bigger muscles and better immunity to improved sex drive, hold onto your wallet!

Vitamin E is a good example of this. Despite its proven benefits, which should be good enough, hucksters continue to market it as a sexual enhancer, which is balderdash. I admit, in my more gullible youth, I avidly read the advertisements about vitamin E. At the tender age of 17, when sex was very much on my mind, I nearly pickled myself with the stuff. At that age, of course, I hardly needed it. It didn't do me any harm, I suppose, but neither did it make me the stud I dreamed of being.

I feel strongly that my medical colleagues are making a grave mistake when they dismiss, out of hand, the potential of alternative treatments. They might be correct to dismiss some approaches when evidence is lacking, but science has a way of proving a lot of us wrong. Even prestigious organizations like the National Cancer Institute are actively investigating alternative approaches. Some, if not most, of these approaches will invariably fall by the wayside. Others will warrant further study, and some, inevitably, will find their ways into the black bag of accepted practice.

In the meantime, how can patients approach these products wisely, with enough knowledge to choose remedies that are likely to work, and enough skepticism to reject those that probably won't? Here are some points to keep in mind.

Any remedy that affects the body in any way is functioning as a drug. "Natural" is meaningless. Any drug, herbal or otherwise, may relieve specific symptoms. It can also cause side effects and interact with other drugs.

Before turning to alternative remedies or treatments, find out what the specific benefits are likely to be. Ask about side effects and interactions. Find out if the treatment interferes with conventional therapy. And finally, see if anything has been published in the medical literature that supports its use.

Ignore testimonials. They're usually made up by marketing departments—and even when they're genuine, there's no guarantee that your experience will be the same as someone else's.

Be suspicious when goods and services sold on the Internet require the completion of a questionnaire. Rest assured that you're being sold something.

The more conditions a specific remedy is said to treat, the less likely it is to be effective.

Run, don't walk, from alternative therapies that promote treatments for cancer or HIV. We know that conventional treatments help. Stick with them.

Finally, let your doctor know when you're using alternative remedies. Herbs, nutritional supplements, and other therapies can interfere with the effects of conventional treatments.

The world of alternative remedies is packed with possibilities for the future. How many cures are waiting to be discovered? I hope there will be many. But until the research has been done, there's simply no way to separate the useful from the fraudulent, the safe from the harmful.

CHAPTER FOUR

"Yesterday I put the mouthwash in the refrigerator and stuck the yogurt under the sink. And last week I forgot it was my sister's birthday. I'm getting worried. Is this how it starts?"

—*Elaine, age 56*

THE MYTH OF AGE-RELATED MEMORY LOSS

Anyone who spends as much time as I do around older adults is going to hear a lot of jokes about memory lapses, those obnoxious, on-the-tip-of-the-tongue moments that proliferate like weeds as we get older. "I'm having an old-timer's moment" is the comment I often hear when someone can't remember the name of a drug they're taking or the title of a recently read novel. I laugh with them because I can relate to the momentary befuddlement you feel when things you should know do a sudden disappearing act. But I also take these comments seriously—not only because memory problems are potentially serious, but because I know that behind the humor there's a lot of unspoken concern. Even run-of-the-mill memory slips, like forgetting where you put the car keys, can't help but raise the frightening specter of Alzheimer's disease, or at least the prospect of decades of mental declines.

I wish I could say that I know better than to worry, but I wouldn't be telling the truth. When I have my own old-timer's moments, I wonder just how bad it's going to get down the road. But I also know, or at least I try to remind myself, that most memory lapses are annoyances, nothing worse. They do get somewhat worse with age, of course. By the time we reach our 40s, we're all having episodes of what doctors call benign forgetfulness. We don't remember names as well. We're not as nimble as we used to be with numbers or other details.

The thing to remember about minor forgetfulness is that it's essentially irrelevant. It isn't an illness, and it doesn't affect your abilities in any meaningful way. Yet there's this pervading sense that older adults are condemned to a lifetime of forgetting names and repeating the same stories again and again. That they'll inexorably reach the stage when they can't mentally function any more.

God knows that Alzheimer's disease and other forms of dementia are frighteningly common. And yes, memory loss is one of the first signs that announce their appearance. But the point that needs to be emphasized, again and again, is that *significant memory loss isn't normal.* It isn't an inevitable consequence of aging. Most of us who are lucky enough to live into our 80s or beyond, assuming that our overall health remains good, will be mentally sharp as a tack.

Frankly, I hate the term "age-related" memory loss. It doesn't make any more sense than talking about age-related cancer or age-related heart disease. Diseases of all sorts get more common with age, but you'll never hear a doctor say, "Oh, you just have normal, age-related cancer." Yet nearly everyone assumes that memory loss and mental declines are somehow an inevitable accompaniment to wrinkles and gray hair. Total nonsense!

WHAT'S NORMAL, WHAT'S NOT

Nearly all of my patients are at least 65 years old, and most are in their 70s, 80s, and 90s. I see a lot of people who have had strokes, or who have Alzheimer's disease or other forms of dementia. Their minds, needless to say, have taken a beating. But I also see a lot of healthy older adults, and believe me, you'd be hard pressed to spot any mental declines. Two patients in particular come to mind. One, a federal judge who was active on the bench right up until his death at age 84, showed absolutely no diminishment in his knowledge and intellectual prowess. The other, a business whiz who built one of the largest department store chains in the United States, always amazed me with his mental speed and grasp of details. Age-related memory loss? Hardly. I had a hard time keeping up with them.

Are these men typical? In many ways, they are. Both stayed in pretty good health throughout their lives. They were lucky enough not to have significant blood vessel disease or other conditions that affect memory or mental functioning. This is a critical point. If you stay physically healthy, there's a very good chance that you'll retain all, or nearly all, of your normal mental abilities. Studies have shown that fully half of those 85 years and older have perfectly normal memories.

But what about the other half? Unfortunately, many of the conditions that affect the mind and memory do get more common with age. About 1 in 20 adults over age 65 has a significant degree of memory loss. Every five years after that, the incidence of memory loss doubles. By age 85, about half of men and women will be having trouble with daily activities, like balancing a checkbook or getting lost in familiar neighborhoods.

The most common cause of memory loss, sad to say, is Alzheimer's disease. Other illness that can cause problems with memory and mental functions are vascular dementia (caused by blocked blood vessels in the brain), high blood pressure, nutritional deficiencies, and depression.

You'll notice that I didn't include aging. To say it yet again, aging doesn't weaken mental vigor. If you're having significant memory lapses—and by significant, I mean memory problems that are seriously affecting your ability to function normally—it's because there's something physically, emotionally, or mentally wrong. Recently, for example, I saw a patient who was having all sorts of memory problems, along with incontinence and problems with balance. He had been diagnosed as having Alzheimer's disease, and his family, needless to say, was falling apart. But when I looked at all of his symptoms, my instincts led me to suspect he had what's called normal pressure hydrocephalus, a condition caused by blocked ventricles, or passageways, in the brain. We brought him in for an MRI (magnetic resonance imaging) scan, and sure enough, that was the problem. He had surgery to unblock the ventricles, and his symptoms disappeared. So much for "natural" memory loss.

One of the most interesting causes of memory problems, and one of the most correctable, is a deficiency of vitamin B12. For some reason, doctors miss this diagnosis all the time. I can't think of anything worse than being told that your mind is going and that you'd better get used to rocking mindlessly on the porch when the solution is as close as the nearest vitamin bottle. The stomach lining of older adults is frequently unable to process vitamin B12, which means that little of the nutrient passes through the small intestine into the bloodstream. About 10% of older adults are deficient in vitamin B12. I've found, when we evaluate people in our memory disorders clinic, that about 17% of patients are either deficient in vitamin B12 or at the very lower limits of the normal range. It's not at all uncommon for their memories to improve once they're given supplemental B12.

There are literally dozens, if not scores, of physical problems that can cause memory to take a nosedive. Some of the most common include:

Depression. It appears to profoundly increase the risk of memory loss. Autopsy studies have found, for example, that depressed people experience brain changes that may affect mental abilities. At the very least, people who are depressed tend to sleep poorly, eat poorly, and generally fail to take care of themselves. It's hardly surprising that a lifetime of depression can compromise health to the degree that memory and mental abilities are affected.

Medications. A great many prescription and over-the-counter drugs, including tranquilizers, sedatives, medications for heart disease, and even antihistamines, can cause memory impairments.

Alcohol. It's among the most common causes of memory problems. The damage may be temporary—people who quit drinking often regain their full memory and cognitive abilities—but it can also result in permanent dementia. Alcohol does indeed fry the brain.

Sleep disorders. They're a common cause of memory problems, mainly because people get so tired and mentally fuzzy that they just can't get their brains into gear. When I evaluate people who complain about lost memory, I always check for sleep apnea, a condition in which breathing frequently stops at night. People with sleep apnea experience dozens or even hundreds of "micro-awakenings," seconds-long sleep disturbances that can cause crushing fatigue the next day. Another sleep disorder, restless legs syndrome, has similar effects. The legs frequently jerk and prevent people from getting the deep sleep that they need to feel alert and refreshed.

These are just a few of the conditions I commonly see that can have significant effects on memory and mental abilities. The darned thing is, they're very easy to treat—but only if doctors suspect them in the first place. I hate to say it, but my medical colleagues, unless they're accustomed to treating older patients, buy into the same myths as everyone else. They're more than willing to dismiss peoples' complaints about memory with that throwaway line, "You're just getting older." Well, *I'm* getting older, and let me tell you, I'm not ready to sit back and accept whatever disabilities come my way. Nor should you. If you're having memory problems—any at all—see your doctor. You may or may not need treatment, but never assume that you're stuck with them. Severe memory lapses are symptoms, not facts of life. Treat the disease, eliminate the symptoms. It's often as simple as that.

THE ALZHEIMER'S PLAGUE

It's impossible to talk about memory problems without discussing Alzheimer's disease. It's far and away the most common cause of memory loss, accounting for about 50% of all cases. This terrible disease occurs when an abnormal protein, amyloid beta, accumulates in the brain. The protein forms clumps that permanently damage or destroy brain cells. A great deal of research is focused on developing drugs that will prevent amyloid beta from accumulating, or that will reduce mind-damaging tangles that are already present. But that's still a long way off. While there are drugs that can slow the progression of Alzheimer's disease, nothing can stop it. There isn't a cure.

The initial symptom of Alzheimer's disease is a loss of short-term memory. As the disease progresses and more areas of the brain are affected, people may experience hallucinations, delusions, and profound personality changes. The time from diagnosis to death averages about 10 years.

We still don't know what causes Alzheimer's disease. There's clearly a genetic link. About half of those with the apolipoprotein E4 gene will go on to develop Alzheimer's. Those with two of the genes—one inherited from each parent—are almost certain to get Alzheimer's disease. For reasons that aren't clear, people who have had head injuries are also more likely to get it. I'm not going to talk a lot about Alzheimer's disease because the treatment options are so limited. But I will say this. Scientists have made a great deal of progress in finding ways to identify the disease at the earliest possible stage, possibly 20 to 30 years before symptoms develop. In the future, when doctors develop drugs that can prevent the protein deposits from accumulating, starting treatments very early has the potential to prevent Alzheimer's disease.

In the meantime, there are a few things you might want to do if Alzheimer's disease runs in your family. The prevention options are highly speculative at this point, but researchers have identified a few factors that might make a difference.

For example, I advise patients to take 400 milligrams of ibuprofen twice daily. Scientists suspect that persistent brain inflammation may cause or contribute to Alzheimer's disease. People who take ibuprofen or other nonsteroidal anti-inflammatory drugs appear to be 50% less likely to get Alzheimer's disease. I also advise people to take 1000 to 2000 IU of vitamin E daily. Like ibuprofen, it reduces brain inflammation by acting as an antioxidant, that is, it "neutralizes" toxic molecules called free radicals, which damage cells in the brain and other parts of the body. While you're taking supplements, add 1000 micrograms of vitamin B12 and 400 micrograms of folic acid to the mix. Taken daily, these nutrients lower levels of an amino acid called homocysteine. Elevated homocysteine has been linked with a higher risk of Alzheimer's disease.

Do make an effort to keep your cholesterol as low as possible, either with dietary changes or, if necessary, by taking a statin drug. There's good evidence that maintaining healthy cholesterol lowers Alzheimer's risk. It's especially important to keep your levels of LDL, the "bad" cholesterol, below 100.

Finally, ask your doctor about supplemental hormones. Research has shown that hormones—estrogen in women and testosterone in men—are potent protectors of memory. Men rarely have low testosterone, but when they do, giving them supplemental amounts makes sense. For women, things aren't quite this straightforward. Doctors used to routinely advise postmenopausal women to take supplemental estrogen. But a large clinical study recently found that women taking a hormone replacement of estrogen plus progesterone had a much higher risk of breast and uterine cancer, blood clots, and heart disease. Because of this study, I only recommend supplemental estrogen for women who have a very strong history of Alzheimer's disease, and who don't have an increased risk of breast cancer or heart disease.

PROTECTING MIND AND MEMORY

With improvements in medical care along with lifestyle factors, such as eating healthier diets and not smoking, people are living longer than ever before. The brain, some experts believe, simply isn't designed to stay healthy for so many years.

Use It or Lose It: Lessons from the Nun Study

We know, however, that there are a number of very practical ways to preserve memory and improve mental functioning and possibly—though this is far from certain—prevent Alzheimer's disease. We're all familiar with the expression, "Use it or lose it." Compelling new research suggests that the brain, like any other part of the body, stays healthier the more it's exercised. One of the most exciting pieces of research in recent years is the elegantly designed Nun Study. Dr. David Snowden and his colleagues at the University of Kentucky followed 678 nuns over a number of years. One goal of the research was to determine how factors such as education and mental activity affect memory as well as the incidence of Alzheimer's disease. The researchers found that nuns with the most education were the ones with the lowest risk of Alzheimer's disease. Nuns who stayed mentally active—by doing research or learning languages, for example—also were more likely to stay healthy and retain robust memories.

What made this study unique is that all of the nuns, regardless of their backgrounds or education levels, had very similar environments. They ate the same foods, had identical access to health care, and maintained the same lifestyles. Because of this, the researchers were able to eliminate "confounding variables" that might explain why some women maintained better memories than others. The study clearly showed that learning and mental activity throughout life is one of the best ways to ensure mental independence in later years.

Reading, Writing, and Arithmetic

I've found myself advising more and more older patients to read books, write letters, learn a foreign language, or do anything else that keeps their minds busy. The Nun Study clearly showed, for example, that women who from an early age were able to write complex sentences, often with excellent prose, were less likely to develop Alzheimer's disease than those who wrote simpler sentences. The researchers also found that women who were read to from an early age were more likely to stay mentally healthy well into their 80s and beyond. The message to me seems very clear: Read a lot (and encourage your children and grandchildren to read). Do crossword puzzles. Take classes at senior centers or community colleges. The more you challenge your brain, the healthier your brain is going to be because you'll constantly be forming additional neural connections. Even if you do develop memory-damaging illnesses at a later time, you'll have a larger reserve of brain cells to help you stay mentally sharp.

Obviously, there's no guarantee that being a lifelong learner will provide 100% protection. We've all known educated adults who developed Alzheimer's disease, or at least profound memory problems, in their later years. And yet, I can't help but believe that their mental activities kept them healthier than they otherwise would have been.

Here's an interesting story that illustrates my point. One of my patients, an 84-year-old woman, was recently diagnosed with Alzheimer's disease. She was a university professor who stayed in the classroom until she was 79. After that, she worked as a tutor until she was 83. The woman has two sisters, both of whom were diagnosed with Alzheimer's disease in their early 70s. We did genetic tests on all three of them. The two sisters who developed Alzheimer's at an earlier age had a single copy of the apolipoprotein E4 gene. The sister who got the disease later in life, the university professor, had two copies of the gene. Her risk for getting Alzheimer's was much higher than her sisters,' yet she was 14 years older than they were at the time of diagnosis. I can't swear that education and a lifetime of mental challenges played a role in forestalling the disease, but it's a reasonable guess. Neither of her sisters, I should add, ever attended college. Both retired early, and both developed Alzheimer's at a much earlier age.

My patients often ask if there are any mental exercises or techniques that will protect their memories. I don't think there are. The main thing is to stay mentally active, and everyone does this in different ways. But if you're already having memory problems, however minor, there are a number of ways to help prevent them from interfering with your life. For example:

Chunk information. No one can remember large blocks of information unless they're somehow organized into smaller pieces. This is why phone numbers are split into two chunks, three numbers followed by four. You can use this technique with anything. When you're going shopping, for example, you'll remember things better if you mentally divide them into categories: produce, meats, dairy, and so on.

Use mental pictures. Form images in your mind of things you want to remember. I do this sometimes because I'm absolutely terrible with names. Suppose I meet someone named Nancy. I might form a mental picture of the cartoon character. The image in my mind's eye will make it easier to remember her name the next time we meet.

Make mental connections. In other words, link things you want to remember with something you already know. Suppose you want to memorize a phone number that starts with "123." Link it to something you're familiar with—the expression "1-2-3-go," for example.

Write things down. This isn't exactly a memory trick, but it's the best way I know to keep from forgetting things. I love those yellow sticky notes because I can put reminders to myself wherever I think I'll see them. Besides, the act of writing things down seems to make them easier to remember—even when I forget to look at the notes!

I've talked quite a bit about the apparent benefits of education, writing, and generally engaging the mind. I think it's worth emphasizing that it doesn't matter all that much what you do, as long as you stay active and involved in life. I'm not aware of any research that suggests that retirement is bad for your health. That said, the evidence is quite clear that people who continue to stay active tend to be physically healthier and mentally more agile than those who do nothing more challenging than watching the grass grow.

One of my best friends is the head of a major foundation—at age 85. Every morning, he stands in front of the mirror and asks himself what he plans to learn that day. Believe me, this guy has more energy than I do, and I'm sure his memory is at least as good as, if not better than, mine. I can't argue with evidence like that. I encourage many of my patients to go back to school and continue their educations, and many of them do. One went on to receive a doctorate in physics when he was in his late 70s. Talk about exercising the mind!

Incidentally, mental activity by itself may be a good thing, but there's increasing evidence that physical activity may be equally important at reducing the risk of memory disorders. Studies have shown that people who are physically active are about 30% less likely to get Alzheimer's disease than those who are sedentary. Even in those who already have Alzheimer's, starting an exercise program appears to slow the rate at which memory declines.

GOOD HEALTH, GOOD MEMORY

I hope I've made it clear that significant memory problems are *always* caused by pathology—abnormalities in the body that affect blood flow, the health of brain cells, and so on. The causes of some of these conditions, such as Alzheimer's, are still a mystery, but many others are well known. My advice is simple: If you have any degree of memory loss, and if it's getting worse over time, get a checkup. There's almost certainly something going on. Insist on an answer. Don't let your doctor minimize your complaints by telling you that it's normal and you should get used to it. Remember, benign forgetfulness—the very minor memory loss that we all experience eventually—should have little or no impact on your daily life. Anything worse than this is caused by something, and it's up to your doctors to figure out what that something is.

It's not enough, incidentally, to take your health seriously only when memory problems start cropping up. A lot of the conditions that affect memory can take years or even decades to cause symptoms. By that time, some of the damage could be permanent. I tell my patients—and I wish that all doctors would do the same—that there are a handful of things they should be doing to protect their minds and memory.

My first piece of advice, and arguably the most important, is to keep your blood pressure healthy. High blood pressure vastly increases the risk of stroke, which in turn can cause vascular dementia. Even pressure in the high-normal range can damage tiny blood vessels in the brain. There's also some evidence that high blood pressure aggravates memory loss in those with Alzheimer's disease. You should be getting your blood pressure checked every time you see your doctor. If the numbers are creeping up, bring them down fast. Blood pressure can almost always be kept in a healthy range with diet and exercise, and, when necessary, with pressure-lowering drugs.

While you're getting your blood pressure checked, ask your doctor to run the necessary tests to check for diabetes or deficiencies of vitamin B12 or thyroid hormone. The thyroid check is especially important. Thyroid deficiencies are very common in those 70 years and older, and forgetfulness is one of the most common symptoms.

One thing you can do on your own is to take a baby aspirin daily. Low-dose aspirin reduces the activity of platelets, cell-like structures in blood that promote the formation of blood clots. These clots have a tendency to drift into the tiny blood vessels in the brain. If they jam a blood vessel, they starve the brain of blood and cause a stroke.

Make sure your cholesterol is low. Studies have shown a link between high cholesterol and Alzheimer's disease. Because of this, lowering cholesterol in my patients is a particularly high priority. Vitamin B12 and folic acid supplements are also of great value, because they lower homocysteine, which may also reduce the risk of Alzheimer's

Another thing you should do, if you're active in the dating scene, is practice safe sex by using condoms. No kidding. Two sexually transmitted diseases, HIV (the virus that causes AIDS) and syphilis, are on the rise in older adults, and both can result in memory loss.

Finally, do what you can to keep stress under control. In a way, I hate giving this advice because we're all subjected to stress on a daily, if not hourly, basis, and there's no way to avoid it. Telling people to avoid stress is like telling them to avoid air or sunshine. Still, staying calm and tranquil is among the most important things you can do. We know that people who successfully manage stress—by exercising regularly, doing yoga, or practicing meditation, for example—are much less likely to experience depression or get a stroke or heart attack. They're also—no surprise here—less likely to experience memory problems as they get older.

SHOULD YOU HAVE YOUR MEMORY TESTED?

Many of my patients, including those who are completely healthy, are almost desperate to know just how good, or bad, their memories are. No matter how much I reassure them that we all forget things from time to time, and that the types of memory lapses they describe are entirely normal, they're never convinced. And I have to say, I'm sympathetic. I know that when I first started forgetting things, way back in my 40s, I was a bit perturbed. Was I losing my grip? Getting Alzheimer's? I really could have used some reassurance—and I'm the doctor!

In any event, there are a number of ways to test memory, and to check for underlying conditions that might be causing problems. When my patients won't accept my reassurances that they're almost certainly fine, I sometimes give them a simple, office-based screening test called Mini-Mental State Examination (MMSE). It's really not sensitive enough to detect very early problems. Nor can it determine who's at high risk for getting memory problems in the future. Still, it's a useful way to detect memory loss that may be starting to affect someone's life.

I can think of two circumstances in which the test is useful. One is to detect early memory loss that might be caused by physical problems that are easily corrected. The other reason is to detect very early signs of Alzheimer's disease. Until recently, there wouldn't have been much use in performing the test to check for Alzheimer's because there wasn't much we could do in the way of treatment. This has changed in the last few years because we now have drugs that can slow the development of Alzheimer's disease. As a result, more and more doctors are using the test to identify those who either fall at the very lower limits of the normal range, or who have a barely identifiable problem. This kind of early memory loss, called minimal cognitive impairment, is a real warning sign. People who have it have a 40% chance of developing additional memory loss within the year. The research is still fairly new, but there's some evidence that treating people aggressively at this very early stage can help prevent more serious memory problems later.

If someone tests positive for minimal cognitive impairment, the next step is to do a complete medical workup to figure out what's going on. We'll often use MRI or PET scans, which can detect early signs that may be Alzheimer's disease. If someone does appear to have Alzheimer's, we usually give them one of three similar drugs: Aricept, Exelon, and Reminyl. They block an enzyme that breaks down acetylcholine, a brain chemical that allows neurons to communicate. When acetylcholine levels fall, memory loss quickly gets worse. People who take these drugs may have some improvement in memory, but their main use is to slow the rate of further memory declines. Recent studies show that people with Alzheimer's disease who take these drugs may gain, on average, two and a half years of living independently.

The research suggests, but it is by no means certain, that giving these drugs at the earliest possible time will provide the most benefits. Patients who take these drugs are often advised to take ibuprofen, folic acid, and vitamins E and B12, as well.

Of course, many of the patients whom I test for minimal cognitive impairment turn out to be fine. Hearing this news certainly helps them sleep better at night, and I can't find any fault with that. If nothing else, it gives me an opportunity to talk to them about what's normal and what's not, and to encourage them to do all of the little things, like eating well and managing their blood pressure, that can prevent memory problems from getting started.

Sometimes the test does reveal memory loss, and the diagnosis may turn out to be Alzheimer's disease. It's the worst kind of news for patients and their families. I do my best to reassure them by explaining that we now have drugs to treat it, and that the disease may take as long as 15 years to progress to an advanced stage. Even to my ears, however, the words ring a little hollow. We're a long way from finding a truly effective treatment for Alzheimer's disease, and families who face it are in for a long, hard journey.

What about the future? I am confident that within my lifetime we'll unlock the secrets of Alzheimer's disease—that we'll be able to prevent it, cure it, or both. In the meantime, it's up to all of us, patients and doctors, to make the extra effort to keep our minds and bodies strong. The truth is, many of the things that we suspect can lower Alzheimer's risk, like getting enough folic acid and vitamin E, and always keeping the mind active and engaged, are the same ones that prevent other types of memory problems. The brain, like every other part of the body, is made up of cells. Keeping these cells healthy—by exercising regularly, eating nutritious foods, not smoking, and so on—should always be a priority. The great thing about lifestyle changes is that they're cheap, they don't have side effects, and you don't need a doctor to prescribe them. And for now, they're by far the most effective way to keep your mind sharp, no matter how old you are when you start.

CHAPTER FIVE

"Every time I see my other doctor, I get another prescription.
First he prescribed metoprolol for my high blood pressure, but
then I got depressed, and so he started me on Prozac. But then
I couldn't sleep, so he prescribed this other antidepressant,
lorazepam. That made me woozy and dizzy, and that's when I
fell and broke my ankle." — *Enid, age 57*

YOU DON'T NEED
ALL THOSE PILLS

I prescribe a lot of drugs. I mention this right away because I don't want to give the impression in the pages that follow that I'm in any way opposed to the sensible use of medications. When patients come to me with serious or not-so-serious problems—depression, insomnia, high blood pressure, constipation, headaches, you name it—I reach for the prescription pad unless there's a compelling reason not to.

I take my hat off to the marvelous research chemists in the nation's pharmaceutical industries. The drugs they've created are among the main reasons that Americans are living longer than ever before. Some of our greatest health threats, such as hypertension and elevated cholesterol, can be almost wholly managed with the appropriate medications.

The hormonal deficiencies that cause diabetes and hypothyroidism are readily corrected with synthetic hormones. Whatever health problem you can think of, there is probably a host of drugs that can help.

Yet I get discouraged when I see my medical colleagues, who are just as influenced by slick marketing campaigns as everyone else, handing out handfuls of drugs without fully considering the implications. We Americans are pretty much pickled in medications—often with great benefit, but too often with great harm. People are given the wrong drugs more often than you might think. Doctors recommend new and "improved" drugs that are no more effective (and much more expensive) than their older counterparts. We spend a hefty percentage of our time treating symptoms caused not by diseases, but by the drugs we hand out with such abandon.

OVERMEDICATION OF THE ELDERLY

I'm aware of two recent studies that suggest that 20 to 30% of adults over age 65 are taking one or more medications that they absolutely shouldn't. Tranquilizers and sleeping pills are two classes of drugs that come to mind, but there are many others. What some of my colleagues don't realize—and what pharmaceutical representatives certainly don't emphasize in their sales pitches—is that older adults respond to drugs in dramatically different ways than younger folks.

When you take a drug, the active ingredients are broken down, or metabolized, by the liver and kidneys. In other words, the active ingredients become inactive fairly quickly. In older patients, however, this process is greatly slowed. Unless doctors take this into account when prescribing medication doses or frequency of doses, older patients are likely to have unsafe concentrations of active drugs circulating in their bodies. This a problem by itself, and it's compounded by the fact that older adults have an increased sensitivity to drug effects. An antihistamine that only causes mild drowsiness in someone in their 30s, for example, can cause profound fatigue or disorientation in someone in their 70s.

Forget the obvious dangers, like falling asleep at the wheel. Older adults whose physical reflexes are slowed by medications have a high risk of breathing food or fluids into the lungs, a common cause of life-threatening pneumonia. Confused and disoriented patients don't eat properly, which can lead to dehydration and malnutrition. They also have a disproportionate number of household accidents because walking and balance are impaired.

There are a handful of drugs (see the chart on page 104) that, in my opinion, should never be prescribed to those 65 years and older. I'm not alone in this opinion. The dangers of these drugs in elderly populations have been very widely reported. And yet, doctors continue to prescribe them—in part, I think, because the majority of drug studies are performed on younger adults, and doctors don't realize that the risk-benefit ratios change dramatically when you're dealing with older adults.

Any drug has the potential to cause side effects, but the risks skyrocket when people take multiple drugs at once. In fact, most iatrogenic diseases—that is, illnesses that are caused by medical treatments—stem from the use of multiple medications, or polypharmacy.

The Risks of Polypharmacy

Polypharmacy means that someone is taking four or more prescription or over-the-counter drugs, any one of which may interact with any of the others. If people had only one doctor, someone who kept track of all the drugs they're taking, the risks could be readily managed. But most of us, as we get older, have many doctors. You might see one specialist who manages your arthritis, another who keeps an eye on your diabetes, another who tracks your heart and blood pressure, and so on. Do you really think that each of these doctors is aware of all the drugs being prescribed by the others? Not a chance.

The more drugs you take, the greater the risk of side effects. In fact, the risk of drug complications is six times higher in those who are taking six or more medications than it is in those who are taking only one. As the list of medications gets longer, so do risks of ill effects. Among adults who are taking eleven or more drugs daily, the risk of adverse reactions approaches 100%. About 26% of hospital admissions are due to drug-related illnesses. In the United States, drug-related deaths rank in the top six of all causes of in-hospital deaths. Drug-related complications took 106,000 American lives in the year 2000.

In our clinic, at least 40% of new patients are taking six or more prescription drugs, and about half of these are taking ten or more. That's a lot of drugs! Especially when you consider that a lot of these patients are also taking over-the-counter or alternative remedies. I have to admit, I love these patients because their problems are often so easy to treat. More times than I can count, the symptoms that brought them to my office—fatigue, dizziness, sexual problems, whatever—disappear when I analyze their medications and shift them to a more sensible, and age-appropriate, treatment plan.

Not that long ago, I saw a man with an alarming array of symptoms. He was suffering from severe fatigue and high blood pressure. He had constipation and indigestion. His memory was shot, he was having hallucinations, and he kept falling down. He had also lost 20 pounds in six months. That's worrisome in anyone, and downright scary in someone 70 years or older. As I always do, I started out by investigating his drug history, and man, I couldn't believe it! He was taking no fewer than fifteen drugs. None of his doctors had bothered to figure out whether drugs, rather than diseases, were causing his symptoms.

I won't bore you with the endless clinical details. The upshot was that I decided to take him off as many of the medications as possible. It wasn't as hard as you might think. I talked to his cardiologist, who admitted that he had prescribed Digoxin and Lasix for a single episode of heart failure that had occurred 10 years earlier. I decided that he probably didn't need to be taking Ativan, a habit-forming antianxiety medicine, and he certainly didn't need to be taking drugs for constipation and indigestion. I saw him almost daily for a month, and the improvements, once he got all those drugs out of his system, were dramatic. In fact, this 79-year-old, surrounded as he was by medical specialists with prescription pads, turned out to be essentially normal. He didn't even have high blood pressure. Apparently, that was just another drug-related side effect.

Snowballing Side Effects

This is a good example of what happens with "cascade prescribing"—giving patients one or more drugs to treat complications caused by other drugs. It happens all the time, and there's nothing wrong, in principle, with using drugs to treat drug-related complications. But it has a way of snowballing, especially when doctors don't realize that the problems they're treated are drug-related. You'd think that doctors would periodically re-evaluate patients to make sure that they're getting appropriate doses of drugs, or that they actually need all the drugs they're taking. But it happens less often than you might think. When confronted with a new symptom, doctors reflexively do what they're trained to do: write another prescription.

I recently read a fascinating case report in a medical journal. It described an 82-year-old man who fell into a coma and was admitted to the hospital. Medical investigators who later put the pieces together realized that the man's symptoms were entirely due to drugs prescribed in a cascade fashion.

• The problems started when his family doctor gave him Vioxx for joint pain.

• Two months later, his cardiologist noted that he had high blood pressure, a side effect of Vioxx. He was given a blood pressure-lowering drug called metoprolol.

• Three months later, he was profoundly depressed, a side effect of metoprolol. A psychiatrist prescribed Prozac. The problem with Prozac is that it sometimes causes insomnia.

• Back to his family doctor. He was advised to take Ambien and Benadryl to help him sleep. Unfortunately, taking these drugs in combination can cause hallucinations. The man's family, in an absolute panic, called the psychiatrist, but they forgot to mention that the family doctor had added these two drugs to his daily regimen.

• The psychiatrist blamed Prozac for the hallucinations. He told the man to quit taking it, and gave him Haldol for the hallucinations.

On and on it went, until the poor fellow was rushed to the emergency room. His recovery, once he was taken off this witches' brew of pharmaceuticals, was almost miraculous. Of course, he was lucky to survive the ordeal.

This might sound like an extreme case, and it is. But drug interactions are a lot more common than you might think, and certainly more common than doctors like to admit. You can't really blame individual doctors. Yes, they should spend more time evaluating the drugs their patients take. Yes, they should be a little less eager to reach for the prescription pads. But our current medical system requires patients to see a great many doctors. There may or may not be a supervising physician who keeps an eye on what the others are doing. The doctors see too many patients and they're rushed for time. Mistakes are all but inevitable.

RISING DRUG COSTS

In 2001, Americans spent $116 billion on prescription drugs—more than double the amount spent in 1993. By 2010, the number will more than double again. The population is getting older, and with advancing age comes a multitude of health problems that require more and more drugs to treat. About 12% of Americans are over age 65, yet they consume 36% of all prescription drugs. The cost of medications is rising much faster than the rate of inflation, a huge problem for those whose insurance plans, such as Medicare, don't cover drugs. The average retiree spends an incredible 19% of income on medications. The problem is even worse for those who depend solely on Social Security: 27% of their disposable income is spent on medications. A recent study found that older adults without drug insurance coverage are fifteen times less likely to take the drugs they need than those who are insured. They simply can't afford it.

Doctors rarely think about the costs of the drugs they prescribe. If anything, they tend to prescribe drugs that are backed by expensive marketing campaigns—which is to say, the newest and most expensive. Every day, physicians are visited by drug sales representatives. You would think that doctors would be inclined to trust their scientific training more than marketing claims, but that's rarely the case. Studies suggest than more than 70% of physicians find the information provided by

DRUGS THAT SHOULDN'T BE USED IF YOU'RE 65 OR OLDER

Medication	What It Does	Side Effects
Diphenhydramine (Benadryl)	Sedative, antihistamine	Confusion, memory loss, increased risk of falls.
Triazolam (Xanax)	Sedative, tranquilizer	Severe confusion, amnesia, bizarre behavior, or agitation. It's 100 times more likely to cause side effects than related drugs.
Chlordiazepoxide (Librium), diazepam (Valium),	Sedative, tranquilizer	Memory loss; confusion; increased risk of falls, fractures, and traffic accidents.
Cimetidine (Zantac)	Antacid	Confusion.
Pentazocine (Talwin)	Analgesic	Hallucinations and psychiatric disturbances.
Chlorpropamide	Diabetes treatment	Facial flushing, rashes, severe reductions in blood sugar.
Meperidine (Demerol)	Analgesic	Severe confusion, nausea, agitation.
Meprobamate (Miltown, Equanil)	Tranquilizer	Confusion; hangover effects; increased risk of falls, fractures, and traffic accidents. Addictive.
Propoxyphene (Darvon)	Analgesic	Confusion, increased risk of falls and fractures. Addictive.
Barbiturates	Sedative	Increased risk of falls and fractures. Addictive. Overdose may cause lung failure.
Belladonna (Donnatal), dicyclomine (Bentyl), hyoscyamine (Levsin), propantheline (Pro-Banthine)	Antispasmodic	Dry mouth, difficulty urinating, sedation, and confusion. May cause irregular heart rates.

drug salesmen to be of real value. Being human, they're also grateful for the free lunches and elaborate dinner meetings sponsored by drug companies. This can't help but influence their prescribing decisions.

Here's something you probably don't know. The vast majority of new drugs that come to market are known as "me too" drugs. They do pretty much the same jobs as older drugs, but because they're new and under patent, they generate mind-boggling profits. For example, many physicians treat mild high blood pressure with calcium channel blockers or ACE inhibitors, relatively new drugs that cost between $2 and $5 daily. Yet most people do just as well when they take the older diuretic hydrochlorothiazide, either alone or in combination with a beta-blocker called atenolol. The combined cost: 12 *cents* a day.

WHEN NEW ISN'T BETTER: LESSONS LEARNED FROM VIOXX AND CELEBREX

There's an old saying in medicine: "When you have a new hammer, everything looks like a nail." Doctors love shiny new gadgets. We get really excited when the pharmaceutical industry comes out with products that promise to solve all our problems. Lulled by persistent salespeople, expensive lunches, and persuasive presentations, we prescribe the heck out of new drugs, even though in the back of our minds there's always the memory of past "miracle" breakthroughs that turned out to be anything but.

As I mentioned before, few new drugs offer significant improvements over older, generic drugs. That's reason enough—were we not so blinded by slick marketing campaigns—to think twice before prescribing them. A more serious issue, one that often gets overlooked in the rush toward new and better, is that new drugs are inherently risky. They haven't been given to millions of people. Doctors don't have decades of experience using them. It's not uncommon for side effects and complications, which appeared to negligible in studies looking at a few thousand people, to come roaring out the door once the drugs enter widespread use. And remember, most drugs are tested in young people, or in healthy older adults without complicating medical problems. Drugs that appear to be very effective in these select groups often turn out to be problematic once they're put to the test in the rather messy real world.

Here's a good example of what happens when we rush too quickly to embrace new drugs. For years, a class of drugs called nonsteroidal anti-inflammatory drugs (NSAIDs) has been the main treatment for arthritis and other chronic causes of joint pain. Drugs in this class, such as aspirin, ibuprofen, naproxen, and indomethacin, reduce inflammation as well as pain. They're effective, but only in high doses—doses that irritate the stomach lining and can cause serious bleeding. Pharmaceutical companies have worked mightily to develop drugs that provide the same benefits as NSAIDs, but without the side effects.

Enter Vioxx and Celebrex. These best-selling drugs belong to a new chemical family called selective COX-2 inhibitors. What makes them special is the "selective" component: They inhibit the inflammation-causing COX-2 enzyme, without suppressing the protective COX-1 enzyme at the same time. These drugs have been promoted for their ability to relieve pain without the gastrointestinal irritation of NSAIDs.

When Celebrex and Vioxx hit the market in 1999, doctors saw them as the new wonder drugs. Their excitement was understandable. Millions of Americans suffer from osteoarthritis. It's the most common disease in older adults, and people who have it depend on anti-inflammatory drugs. For the first time, it seemed, patients with osteoarthritis could effectively treat their symptoms without suffering painful consequences. The drugs were almost instant best-sellers, and have since generated more than $6 billion in revenues.

Have the drugs lived up to their early promise? As so often happens when new drugs take the medical world by storm, the answer would have to be no. COX-2 inhibitors do relieve pain and inflammation. They do cause fewer side effects than traditional NSAIDs. But they're far from being the wonder drugs that doctors anticipated. Recent studies have shown that COX-2 inhibitors are *more* likely than naproxen and other NSAIDs to be linked with heart problems. Unlike NSAIDs, COX-2 inhibitors don't suppress the activity of platelets, cell-like structures in blood that can form clots and increase the risk of heart disease and stroke. People who depend on COX-2 inhibitors for pain relief are five times more likely to have a heart attack than those who take aspirin. People with heart problems who take these drugs may have a greater risk of heart failure. The drugs have also been linked to rises in blood pressure and swelling in the legs or feet.

None of this means that Celebrex and Vioxx aren't perfectly acceptable drugs. They do relieve pain and inflammation in those with osteoarthritis. They appear to be helpful for headache and menstrual pain. In higher-than-normal doses, they've even been found to reduce postoperative pain as well as morphine. But the real question is whether they represent a real breakthrough, and whether they're the best choice for older adults with joint pain.

Maybe not. As I mentioned, people who take COX-2 inhibitors miss out on the heart benefits that they get from aspirin and other NSAIDs. Vioxx and Celebrex do appear to provide superior pain relief, but the difference isn't all that pronounced. Even in the area of side effects, they fall short of their early promise. Many people who take COX-2 inhibitors for joint pain also take aspirin for the heart-healthy benefits—

a combination that produces gastrointestinal side effects at a much higher rate than aspirin alone.

So much for new and improved. Except in rare cases, I advise patients with osteoarthritis to stick with Motrin (ibuprofen) or Tylenol (acetaminophen). I usually start with Tylenol initially—two extra-strength tablets taken three or four times daily. If this doesn't help, they can add 400 milligrams of Motrin twice a day. Most of the time, this provides adequate relief. If it doesn't, I go ahead and recommend that they replace Motrin with a COX-2 inhibitor. In either case, I always encourage people to get plenty of exercise, with or without the help of a physical therapist, and to keep their weight at healthy levels. As is often the case, lifestyle changes often produce better results than the newest "breakthrough" drugs—and they never cause side effects.

DRUGS TO AVOID AT ALL COSTS

So far, I've talked mainly about prescribing habits—the tendency of doctors to prescribe new drugs, or too many drugs, with too little investigation. Now, I'd like to talk about an equally serious problem: the use of drugs that are absolutely inappropriate for people ages 65 and older. As we've seen, elderly adults don't metabolize drugs as efficiently as younger people. They're more sensitive to drugs and more prone to drug-related complications. Doctors who neglect to consider these factors are writing prescriptions for disaster.

Diphenhydramine

I don't worry too much when my patients dip into over-the-counter drugs, but I strongly object when I learn they're taking diphenhydramine. An antihistamine sold under the brand name Benadryl, it's also an active ingredient in a number of pain and cold remedies.

Diphenhydramine is an excellent antihistamine, and it has the added attraction (or side effect, depending on your point of view) of acting as a sedative. For decades, doctors have recommended this drug for allergy symptoms as well as to promote sleepiness. It's so commonly used, in fact, that I have a hard time convincing people how dangerous it can be.

The sedation caused by diphenhydramine can be exceptionally long-lasting, especially in those 65 years and older. People who take it for insomnia often find themselves disoriented, sleepy, and hung over the next day. It can trigger, or at least exacerbate, depression in some people. Research has shown that it can slow reaction times even more than alcohol, substantially increasing the risk of accidents. Don't drive if you're taking diphenhydramine. No kidding, it's dangerous.

Here's a story that should scare anyone. One of my patients was a very healthy 80-year-old. She lived on her own and had few physical problems. Then she came down with a mild upper respiratory infection. The cough was keeping her awake at night, so she decided to take Tylenol PM, a product that contains diphenhydramine and is promoted as a sleep aid. She fell asleep quickly enough, but then woke up at about 2 A.M. I'm not sure what happened next. Maybe she got up to go to the bathroom or get a drink of water. She might have been disoriented or confused. In event, she fell, fractured her hip, and was unable to get up. She lay on the floor, I'm sure more frightened than I care to imagine, until her daughter found her there the next morning at about 9 o'clock.

There's a lot more to the story, none of it happy. Her hip took a long time to heal. She never fully regained her strength or balance. Her confidence was shot. This strong, independent woman was never healthy enough to live by herself again.

Obviously, diphenhydramine may have been just one of many factors that contributed to this dreadful accident. But there's no question that the drug is really too strong and unpredictable in its effects to be a good choice for older adults. I advise almost everyone to avoid it. If you have trouble with allergies, take one of the nonsedating antihistamines. Despite the name, they do have a very slight sedating effect, so you can take them for mild sleeplessness, as well.

Tranquilizers and Sleeping Pills

If you're feeling a little anxious and stressed, you won't have any trouble finding an accommodating doctor who will prescribe a wonderfully calming drug, such as Valium, Librium, Xanax, or Ativan. Having trouble sleeping? Take Halcion, Sonata, or Ambien.

I can think of plenty of occasions when the use of these drugs is appropriate. It's not uncommon, for example, for one of my elderly patients to lose a spouse or sibling. I see no problem with using sedatives to help them cope with stress and anxiety for a few days or weeks. Similarly, insomnia gets more common with age, and people sometimes need medical help to sleep soundly and establish better sleep habits.

But frankly, sedatives and tranquilizers are grossly overused. They aren't particularly good for anyone, and they can be devastating for older adults if they're not used with very careful supervision. The doses that are normally used are much too strong for those 65 years and older. And because older adults require more time to clear the drugs from their systems, blood concentrations can easily rise to toxic levels. Even short-acting sedatives commonly cause some degree of daytime drowsiness. Memory lapses become more pronounced. The risk of falls, perhaps the worst thing that can happen, is greatly increased. Studies have shown, in fact, that the risk of falls *doubles* in those who take benzodiazepines—a chemical class of drugs that includes Valium, Halcion, and Xanax. The drugs also cause measurable declines in mental abilities, and they're addictive in some cases. And yet, my patients almost beg for them. Go figure.

I'm not suggesting that there's a magic cut-off age that determines whether you should or shouldn't take these drugs. If you're 60, 70, or 80, however, do think long and hard before taking them. The long-term negative effects can more than outweigh the temporary benefits. Besides, medications should be the last, not the first, line of treatment for anxiety. Especially because most patients who ask for these drugs don't have significant anxiety—at least, not the kind of anxiety that's seriously affecting their ability to function normally.

The line I usually hear is, "I'm so tense and worried, I really need a Xanax." Well, they might. But I doubt it. Unless you have true anxiety, defined as feeling anxious or worried on most days for a minimum of six months, you probably don't need drugs. Even if you have anxiety, you'll do better in the long run by seeing a therapist and reducing stress by getting more exercise, eating nutritious foods, and so on. Turning to drugs, even those prescribed by a doctor, to control daily stress can be as destructive as turning to alcohol.

I have pretty much the same advice for those who bitterly complain about insomnia. I always ask how tired they are during the day. If they say they aren't particularly fatigued, I tell them not to worry. They're apparently sleeping enough. Those who are fatigued may in fact have insomnia, but drugs should still be the last choice. Nearly everyone will sleep better when they do common-sense things like cutting back on caffeine, exercising more, and perhaps practicing yoga or other stress-reducing techniques.

I don't mean to minimize the impact that insomnia can have on peoples' lives. Anyone who's persistently having trouble sleeping should see a doctor. Insomnia can be caused by a variety of physical problems, a breathing disorder called sleep apnea, for example, or a mysterious condition called restless legs syndrome. It's also possible that the internal body clock isn't working the way it should. What usually happens, though, is that people have a few sleepless nights, then get so worried about it that they're essentially scared into insomnia. Sleeping pills can certainly tide people over for a few days. But to use them routinely? Never.

Anticholinergics

This is a very broad class of medicines that includes antihistamines, antispasmodics, and some antidepressants. Anticholinergic drugs work by reducing the effects of a body chemical called acetylcholine. This has many different effects in the body. For example, reducing acetylcholine causes the bowel to contract less vigorously, which is helpful for irritable bowel syndrome. Those with a type of urinary incontinence called urge incontinence might take anticholinergics to reduce bladder contractions. The anticholinergic properties of antihistamines are what make these drugs useful for reducing allergy symptoms as well as promoting sleepiness.

Two of the most powerful anticholinergic drugs, and the ones that tend to cause the most problems in older adults, are the sedating antidepressants Elavil and Doxepin. They aren't used as much as they used to be, but they're still used too often, in my opinion. People who take them may experience confusion, a very dry mouth, and a significant worsening of memory problems.

Drugs that cause similar problems include those used to treat abdominal cramps (Bentyl, Levsin, Pro-Banthine, Donnatal), some antihistamines (Chlor-Trimeton, Vistaril, Atarax, and Benadryl), and muscle relaxants such as Robaxin, Soma, Paraflex, Skelaxin, and Flexeril.

There are plenty of legitimate uses for these drugs, of course. If there weren't, doctors wouldn't prescribe them and patients wouldn't take them. Elavil, for example, which has fallen out of favor as an antidepressant, is very helpful at reducing nerve pain caused by peripheral neuropathy and shingles. The drugs Ditropan and Detrol are good choices for urinary incontinence, despite their anticholinergic effects. But for the most part, I try to avoid the anticholinergic drugs altogether. When I do prescribe them, I choose the lowest possible dose.

Pain Medications

I'm always amazed that doctors continue to prescribe the painkillers Darvon and Darvocet. But prescribe them they do: Surveys show that up to 6% of older adults take Darvon regularly. These pain relievers do the job, all right, but they're no more effective than plain Tylenol, and they're rife with side effects, especially addiction. I think that's the reason that so many of my new patients almost beg for one or the other of these drugs. I almost never give them—although, to be honest, addiction is the least of my worries. In older adults, narcotics frequently cause confusion or disorientation. The risk of hip fractures is greatly increased in those who take them. And because the drugs are in fact addictive, many people suffer the terrible discomfort of withdrawal when they quit taking them.

Managing pain is always a challenge. The most important principle is that it is much easier to prevent pain than to relieve it. That's why I advise people to take medication before they need it—and to keeping taking more (at the appropriate times) rather than wait for the pain to come back. For most people, taking extra-strength Tylenol three or four times daily is effective. When that doesn't work, I advise them to add one of the NSAIDs, such as ibuprofen or naproxen. A relatively new prescription drug, Ultram, can replace Tylenol for more serious pain. It's as effective as codeine, but causes fewer side effects.

Antibiotics

I debated for a long time before including antibiotics in my list of "shouldn't take" drugs. After all, antibiotics have revolutionized the practice of medicine. Prior to the 1940s, when antibiotics were first developed, millions of Americans died every year from the kinds of simple infections that we treat with a few pills today. Thanks to antibiotics, infant mortality has plunged and our lifespans are much longer than they used to be. And yet, these same drugs, if we keep using them the way we have, are almost certain to put us right back where we started: at the mercy of the germs that surround us.

Here's the problem. Through the process of normal genetic mutations, bacteria gradually become resistant to the drugs used to kill them. Today, more than 80% of the bugs that cause urinary tract infections are no longer sensitive to penicillin. Other drugs still work, but it won't be long before bacteria become resistant to them, as well. This is happening across the spectrum of infectious organisms. The germs that cause some types of pneumonia now respond only to the hardcore (and expensive) antibiotics vancomycin and levofloxacin. About 50% of the bacteria that cause tuberculosis are resistant to the drugs that used to kill them. What happens when these and other organisms develop resistance to all of the available drugs? We'll have a devastating crisis on our hands.

The excessive and unnecessary use of antibiotics is among the main causes of resistance. Doctors readily prescribe them, and patients invariably demand them, for the most minor symptoms. Studies have found that one in seven prescriptions given in outpatient clinics is for an antibiotic to treat upper respiratory infections, acute coughs, bronchitis, or a stuffy nose or sinuses. How stupid can we be? More than 95% of these minor infections are caused by viruses, not bacteria. Antibiotics don't kill viruses, so the drugs can't possibly work. Doctors know this, but they keep prescribing antibiotics because their patients expect it.

Even more alarming is the trend among doctors to prescribe the strongest antibiotics—drugs like clarithromycin, ciprofloxacin, and levofloxacin—when ampicillin and other garden-variety antibiotics work just as well. The stronger, broad-spectrum antibiotics are our last lines of defense against resistant bacteria, yet they're being handed out like candy. It's only a matter of time before bacteria develop resistance. What will we do then?

I get calls every day from patients who demand antibiotics. They don't want to come into the office, mind you. They just want the drugs. "I've been coughing for a week, can you give me an antibiotic?" Or, "I'm going on a cruise, can you write me a prescription just in case I get sick?" And the darned thing is, we write the prescriptions. I suppose it's because writing a prescription makes us feel powerful. We're giving the appearance, at least, that something is being done. It takes less time to write a prescription than to explain, over and over again, why antibiotics probably aren't necessary. We save time, the patient leaves the office happy, and the infection—which probably will go away on its own in any event—does get better.

More and more, I'm refusing to give patients antibiotics unless I'm convinced that they'll make a real difference. This is easier for me than many of my colleagues because I work in a geriatric setting. I typically spend more time with each patient. I'm able to discuss the differences between viral and bacterial infections and help people understand why the drugs aren't necessary. I also point out that there's nothing wrong with "watchful waiting"—withholding treatment for a few days in order to see how the infection does on its own. Studies have shown that when doctors take this approach—talking to patients, watching symptoms closely, and initially withholding drugs—the use of antibiotics can be reduced by 50% without affecting the cure rates.

DON'T LET DRUGS KILL YOU

I've been discussing drugs that, in my view, should almost never be used. But it's also worth mentioning some of the problems that occur when good drugs are used inappropriately. Antibiotics clearly belong in this category. So do many others. The short-acting sleeping pill Ambien, while much safer than some of its predecessors, is well known for causing confusion, along with unnecessary falls, in the elderly. Any drug can be a bad drug if it's not used wisely.

I wish I could say with confidence that doctors are sufficiently aware of the risks of drug therapy, that all prescriptions are written with a judicious consideration of the trade-off between risks and benefits. In the real world of medicine, this is more of an ideal than the reality. Doctors spend precious few minutes with each patient. The sheer volume of new information makes it impossible to keep up with all the latest developments. Doctors may or may not understand that people of different age groups react to drugs differently.

Most drug decisions are often based on handouts from pharmaceutical representatives, or on the information that doctors glean at scientific meetings featuring "expert" testimony, the experts, of course, being doctors who receive generous compensation from drug companies. Drug companies don't deliberately mislead physicians. In most cases, they try to be scrupulous about presenting all the known facts, risks as well as benefits. But they are in the business to make money, and this invariably influences their presentations. Doctors who don't balance drug company perspectives with more objective data are putting their patients at risk.

The bottom line, I'm afraid, is that you can't depend entirely on your doctor to ensure that the drugs you're taking are the best ones for you.

Nor can you trust what you read in the media. New drugs aren't always the best drugs. In fact, the opposite is often true, because new drugs haven't been taken by sufficient numbers of patients for doctors to identify all of the possible side effects or risk factors. A drug that's been on the market for decades is unlikely to have many surprises. You can't say that about a drug that hit the headlines last week.

If you're 65 or older, you have to be especially vigilant. Doctors who see a lot of older patients, such as geriatricians and internists, are well trained in the age-specific guidelines for different drugs. A family practitioner might not be. Regardless of who your primary doctor is, I strongly recommend learning as much as you can about the drugs you're taking. The *Physicians' Desk Reference* (commonly known as "The PDR") is a good starting place. You can also find useful drug information on the Internet. Take the time to learn how the drugs you're taking work. Pay attention to likely side effects in different age groups. Take lots of notes and pester your doctor with questions. You have to protect yourself.

Specifically, here are a few things you'll want to do.

If you're 65 or older, discuss the drugs you're taking with a geriatrician, a specialist in treating older adults.

If you're seeing more than one doctor, ask the one you trust most if he or she will take charge of coordinating all your care. It's essential to have one person, usually an internist or geriatrician, who's watching the big picture. This doctor might agree to review all your prescriptions. At the very least, he or she should periodically review all the drugs that you're taking.

Every time you see a doctor, bring along a list of the drugs you're currently taking, along with the doses. This includes prescription drugs, of course, and also herbs, supplements, or other over-the-counter products. Have the doctor look the list over. Do you need all the drugs? Are the doses correct? Will any of the drugs interact with others?

Be familiar with both the generic and brand names of the drugs you're taking, and make sure you know *why* you're taking them. Not that long ago, I reviewed the drug history of a new patient. She was taking 100 milligrams daily of both amitriptyline and Elavil. What she didn't know—and, apparently, one of her doctors didn't either—was that Elavil is simply the brand name of the drug amitriptyline. She was inadvertently taking a double dose of the same drug.

Buy all your drugs from the same pharmacy. Most pharmacies these days keep computerized records. Your pharmacist might catch potential problems—interactions, inappropriate doses, duplicate drugs, and so on—that your doctor missed.

Follow directions exactly. Read the label every time you take your medication. Take drugs at the proper times and at the proper doses. Many side effects are caused by poor compliance—another way of saying that patients don't follow directions. If you have occasional or frequent problems with memory, enlist a friend or family member who will help you keep tabs on your drug consumption. Medication trays, which allow you to arrange drugs according to the days or times that they're supposed to be taken, can be very helpful.

Keep track of new symptoms as they develop. Write them down. Then ask your doctor or pharmacist if any of the drugs you're taking might be responsible

CHAPTER SIX

*"I feel great, Doctor David! That heart attack was a real
wake-up call. Since the surgery, I'm eating better, and Annie
and I walk every day. I don't have to take anything anymore.
I'm even off that blood pressure medicine."*   —Calvin, age 59

LIFESAVING HEART DRUGS THAT AREN'T USED ENOUGH

s Americans, we're more likely to die from heart disease than
nearly all other diseases combined. About 65% of men and
55% of women in their 60s and older have artery damage
severe enough to be called coronary artery disease. In any given year,
more than a million people have heart attacks, and upward of 400,000
people will die of heart disease. Those are some daunting statistics. You
would think that doctors would be all over this issue—not only looking
for heart disease or heart disease risk factors in older patients, but also
giving the drugs that have been clearly shown to save their lives.

But they're not. *Fewer than half of Americans at risk for heart disease
are getting the drugs that they need.* Maybe it's because doctors are so
busy that they don't take the time to fully analyze their patients' histories

and sort through the dozens of appropriate drugs. Or maybe they're so attuned to acute, treat-them-now conditions that long-term illnesses—the ones that are most likely to kill you—pass beneath the radar. In any event, tens of thousands of people die unnecessarily because they aren't getting the drugs they need.

I recently evaluated a 66-year-old man with recurrent chest pains typical of angina, a potentially dangerous condition in which insufficient blood reaches the heart. He had had a heart attack 10 years ago, which was followed by open heart surgery. As is usually the case, he quit seeing his cardiologist about a year after the surgery. Since then, he's been followed by his family physician. As far as he was concerned, his heart problems were ancient history. His doctor apparently felt the same way. He wasn't giving this guy any of the treatments that he so clearly needed. Don't ask me why. The indications were all there, and it didn't take more than a quick checkup and a couple of simple lab tests to prove it.

His blood pressure was 157/80—not the worst reading, by any means, but definitely on the high side. His total cholesterol was elevated at 260. More worrisome, his levels of HDL (the "good" cholesterol) were extremely low, while his levels of LDL (the "bad" cholesterol") were dangerously high. I ran blood tests for diabetes, and they came back positive.

Forget for the moment that the guy had a couple of undiagnosed conditions that any doctor should have picked up. The fact that he had a history of heart disease, and now had diabetes and elevated blood pressure and cholesterol, meant that he was at very high risk for another heart attack. To put it bluntly, he was a walking time bomb, and no one was doing much about it. I asked him, for example, if he was taking aspirin. Aspirin is essential for someone who's had a heart attack or is at risk for heart disease because it can dramatically reduce the risk of clots that can cut off circulation to the coronary arteries. One of his doctors had suggested aspirin, he admitted, but he quit taking it because it upset his stomach. No one even suggested that he should be taking drugs to lower his blood pressure. His cardiologist did advise him to improve his diet to lower his cholesterol, but he never followed up to see if the diet was working.

Talk about dropping the ball! Any doctor who was serious about saving this man's life would have *insisted*, not "suggested," that he take aspirin daily. The same for lowering cholesterol and blood pressure. I suppose if the poor man had lurched into his doctor's office, clutching his chest and moaning with pain, he would have been rushed into treatment. He might even have gotten some decent counseling about lifestyle changes. But because he generally seemed healthy, no one bothered to predict his likely future—a future that, with his risk factors, was almost certain to include a second heart attack, followed by surgical procedures that he might or might not survive. If anyone was a good candidate for aggressive medical therapy, this guy was definitely it. Yet he wasn't getting it. Why not?

NO ATTENTION TO PREVENTION

Doctors today are incredibly rushed. They only spend about six minutes with each patient—if you're lucky—before rushing to the next appointment. In busy family practices or internal medicine clinics, it's almost impossible for doctors to get to know their patients or fully investigate their medical histories. The best they can hope for is to manage the current crisis, whatever it is. They don't have time to worry about tomorrow or the day after. We all talk about the value of preventive care, but when you spend your entire day putting out fires, tomorrow can always wait.

The problem, of course, is that tomorrow is everything. Heart disease doesn't spring up all at once. It usually accrues over decades, and it can almost always be stopped by identifying and correcting risk factors, such as elevated cholesterol and blood pressure, at the earliest possible time. By the time a patient has symptoms, the damage is already done.

Don't be lulled by promises of high-tech salvation, either. It's true that doctors in the United States have access to state-of-the-art treatments that are the envy of the world. But you can't count on technology to save your life. When it comes to overall health and longevity, the United States isn't even in the top ten worldwide. In fact, patients with heart disease or heart disease risk factors fare a lot better in France, Germany, and other European countries. Not because treatments in these countries are superior, but because they put a lot more emphasis on prevention. They don't wait for heart disease to happen. They treat patients with state-of-the art drugs at the earliest possible times. Their bias is always to treat patients aggressively, but conservatively; invasive procedures are last resorts. In Sweden, for example, cardiologists and cardiac surgeons only perform one angioplasty or open heart surgery for every eight that are done in the United States.

In this country, on the other hand, more than 60% of patients with heart disease who have elevated cholesterol don't get the drugs they need to lower it. Only 30% of those who could benefit from aspirin are taking it. More than half of those with hypertension don't get diagnosed, or treated, for years. And less than 40% of those who have had a heart attack or are known to have heart disease are taking either a beta-blocker or an ACE inhibitor, drugs that are essential for reducing the risk of heart failure, a second heart attack, or sudden death.

The lack of attention to preventive strategies isn't entirely the fault of the health care system. Anyone with even a passing interest in nutrition and health knows what needs to be done to control the main heart disease risk factors. Take the patient I discussed earlier. He was hardly naïve. He knew that he had to lower his cholesterol, and he easily could have asked his doctor to schedule tests to track how well he was doing. Similarly, he knew that his high-stress job as an investment banker wasn't doing him any good, but he never seriously considered a career change or looked into ways to keep his stress at manageable levels. Prevention is everyone's business. When doctors don't take it seriously, it's up to patients to shake them up.

Anyway, back to my patient. Once I knew he had diabetes, which vastly increases the risk of heart disease, I referred him to a cardiologist, who confirmed that he had coronary artery disease. Surgery certainly would have been a reasonable approach, but the patient didn't want it. He was sufficiently rattled by mortality statistics to take lifestyle changes seriously. He agreed to take aspirin daily, and so far he's been rigorous about exercising and practicing stress reduction. At the same time, I gave him the drugs he should have been taking all along: a statin drug to lower cholesterol, and a beta-blocker and ACE inhibitor to lower blood pressure and prevent future heart attacks. Because his coronary arteries were so damaged by the time I saw him, his risk for a second heart attack will always be somewhat elevated. But he's clearly doing a lot better than he was. His cholesterol and blood pressure have stayed in a healthful range, his diabetes is controlled by diet alone, and he's had no chest pain for three years.

THE BEST DRUGS FOR PREVENTING HEART ATTACKS

In the following pages, you'll notice a number of references to "miracle" drugs. I use the term advisedly. I do think there are a handful of drugs that can truly work miracles in some patients, and it's clear that these drugs are used a lot less often than they should be. But no drug is perfect, and science changes all the time. Treatments that seem optimal today may turn out to be less than ideal, or even hazardous, a few years from now. (Consider the latest headlines on hormone replacement therapy after menopause. For decades, we were so sure of the benefits of estrogen and other hormones that we did everything but dispense them with a hose. Only recently has the use of these drugs been called into question. Yes, they're effective for treating menopausal discomfort, and they do help prevent age-related bone loss. But a large recent study found that hormone replacement therapy increases the risk of heart attacks, blood clots in the legs, and breast cancer. Those of us who enthusiastically recommended these drugs were, to put it mildly, wrong.)

So keep this proviso in mind: The drugs I'm about to discuss show a great deal of promise. Some of them prevent heart attack and heart failure. They may reduce deposits of cholesterol in the arteries. They have positive effects on memory and diabetes, and they may play a role against cancer. Side effects are often an issue, of course, but these are generally minor and easy to control. Any doctor who sees patients with risk factors for heart disease should strongly consider using one or more of these drugs. Failure to use them—or at least to consider them—is just bad medicine. Indeed, if you're a candidate for one of these drugs, and your doctor hasn't written the prescription, I'd advise you to demand why not.

The Amazing Statins

The best drugs for lowering cholesterol, and by far the most prescribed, are the statins. Drugs in this class, such as Mevacor, Zocor, Pravachol, Lipitor, and Lescol, suppress an enzyme called HMG-CoA reductase. Suppressing this enzyme inhibits the production of cholesterol in the liver. These are truly remarkable drugs, in part because they dramatically lower levels of harmful LDL cholesterol without significantly depressing the beneficial HDL. One large study of 20,000 high-risk patients found that those who took statins and achieved a target LDL level below 100 were able to reduce their risk of heart attack and stroke by 30%. That's impressive! The drugs are especially good because they appear to work in all populations: women as well as men, the elderly, and those with diabetes. Statins even appear to reduce the risk of heart disease in those with normal cholesterol.

More than a few doctors have said that the statins are so effective, and so safe for most people, that they should be added to the nation's drinking water. Studies suggest, in fact, that 50,000 lives could be saved for every 10 million high-risk patients who take these drugs. The current cholesterol guidelines suggest that 36 million Americans are good candidates for statin therapy. Yet despite the clear benefits of these drugs, and their outstanding safety profiles, only about 15 million people—less than half of those who are eligible—are currently taking them. In some cases, this is because people have never had a cholesterol screening. The drugs are expensive, and that can be a factor. And in a lot of cases, doctors simply don't push them hard enough.

The bias of our medical system is to focus on treatment rather than prevention. Patients with high cholesterol who have had heart attacks will very likely be given a statin. But what about the millions of people who could benefit from primary prevention—those without coronary artery disease who are generally in good health, but who happen to have elevated cholesterol that doesn't respond to diet or exercise? They're not getting the drugs, and they should be. Research has shown with a fair degree of certainty that healthy people can benefit from statins. One study, for example, looked at more than 6500 men and women with elevated LDL cholesterol. Those who took the statin lovastatin for more than five years had reductions in LDL of more than 25%, and their heart attack risk dropped 40%.

Additional Benefits of Statins. While the main benefit of the statins is lowering cholesterol, they have other beneficial functions that still aren't clearly understood. As I mentioned, people with normal cholesterol who take statins have a lower risk of heart disease. Since cholesterol isn't the issue in these cases, something else must be happening in the body. The drugs have been shown to have distinct anti-inflammatory properties. A decade ago, this would have elicited a shrug from cardiologists, but the evidence is now clear that inflammation in the coronary arteries contributes to heart disease and may even precipitate heart attacks. Inflammation tends to occur in areas with thick layers of plaques—fatty deposits that form in sections of the arteries. The inflammation seems to act as a magnet for platelets, those sticky, cell-like structures that aid in clotting. Clots are good when you cut your finger, but not when they form inside the blood vessels. Clots have a nasty habit of breaking away from artery walls, drifting into narrow sections of blood vessels, and abruptly blocking the flow of blood. Stopping inflammation with statins is one way to help prevent clots from forming.

This by itself would be reason enough to take statins, but the drugs do more. They stimulate the production of nitric oxide in the endothelial cells that line the blood vessels. Nitric oxide prevents arterial spasms and promotes better blood flow. Statins also appear to stimulate the production of new blood vessels in areas where the heart isn't getting enough blood.

Here are a few additional reasons I wish doctors would take these drugs more seriously. There is rather compelling evidence that they may help delay the onset of Alzheimer's disease. One study found that older women with elevated cholesterol who took statins for four years experienced the same rates of memory loss as those with normal cholesterol. Among women with high cholesterol who didn't take the drugs, the risk of significant memory loss was increased 77%. As far as I'm concerned, the evidence is sufficiently strong that I routinely recommend statins for people with elevated LDL cholesterol who also have a family history or other risk factors for developing Alzheimer's disease.

Now, the really exiting news. The research is far from conclusive, but a number of studies suggest that statins may play a powerful role in preventing cancer. Canadian researchers, for example, found that the risk of developing any cancer was 28% lower in those taking statins than in those taking placebos. In another study, this one involving 8000 women, statins appeared to dramatically reduce the risk of breast cancer. In the study group, 191 women developed breast cancer, but only three of them were taking statins. So far, we can only guess why the drugs are beneficial. It's possible that they somehow modulate the effects of estrogen in the body. Or maybe they reduce the carcinogenic effects of inflammation or declines in immune function. It's too early to say with certainty that statins prevent cancer, and I won't recommend them for this until more is known. But it's nice to know that people who take these drugs for cholesterol control may be getting an unexpected bonus at the same time.

Who Should Take Statins? So who should be taking statins? The optimal time to start treatment is still controversial, but a few things seem clear. People with familial hypercholesterolemia—a genetic condition that results in high cholesterol regardless of lifestyle factors—should always be treated with statins. Most men get heart attacks at age 40 and beyond; women are more at risk after menopause. My feeling is that men should have cholesterol screenings at age 40. Women can wait a little longer, until about age 45 or 50. If the numbers are high, it's fine to try to bring them down with diet, exercise, and other lifestyle approaches. If this doesn't work, by all means, bring on the statins. Their use is certainly advised when LDL is higher than 160, or when levels of protective HDL are relatively low.

Okay, now for some caveats. The statins aren't a one-time thing. Once you start taking them, you have to take them for life. When you consider the long-term costs as well as the inconvenience, that's no small thing. There's also a health issue involved: People who abruptly stop taking the drugs have an increased risk of a heart attack. Another drawback to statins is that they may cause muscle cramps. The cramps are usually minor, but in rare cases they may progress to severe muscle damage. (This complication occurred frequently with a statin called Baycol, which was pulled off the market in the mid-1990s.) Statins have also been known to cause liver problems. It doesn't happen often, but it's common enough that you'll need regular liver tests once you start taking them.

Overall, however, the statins are remarkably safe. Side effects do occur, but no more often—and usually much less—than with other drugs. Their benefits are so pronounced, and so varied, that I wouldn't be surprised if their officially recommended uses soon extend way beyond cholesterol control. In the next few years, when the original patents expire, you'll see generic versions of these drugs, which means the costs will plummet.

I do hope that more and more doctors see the light and start prescribing these drugs more liberally. Millions of patients would benefit immeasurably—from lower cholesterol, less risk of heart disease and stroke, and possibly less cancer or Alzheimer's disease. Unless new research proves me wrong, I have to say that the statins are some of the most amazing drugs to come along in a long time. They're not, needless to say, a substitute for healthy living. More than a few of my patients have given little prayers of thanks to drugs that appear to give them the liberty to wolf down high-fat meals, keep smoking, and generally live lives of high debauchery. Hey, they're not *that* good. The benefits of the statins, however dramatic, can't compete with the benefits of healthful living. But the evidence is persuasive that combining statins with good habits can allow you to live longer and with fewer diseases than you would without them. That's a pretty good definition of "miracle drug," don't you think?

Aspirin: An Inexpensive Miracle

The evidence is absolutely conclusive: Aspirin taken daily (or every other day) dramatically reduces the risk of heart attacks. The American Heart Association advises older adults to take one baby (81.5 milligrams) aspirin daily. Personally, I recommend taking an adult (325 milligrams) aspirin because larger doses have additional benefits besides protecting the heart.

For the life of me, I can't figure out why more doctors aren't advising—no, *telling*—their patients to take aspirin. Currently, less than 20% of people 50 and older are taking aspirin daily for preventive purposes, and they're the ones who need it most. Partly, I suppose, it's because people who are in good health assume that they're always going to be that way. Also, aspirin is well known for causing stomach upset, and some people are convinced it causes bruises. Aspirin is hard on the stomach, but not at the doses we're talking about. I've only occasionally encountered people who can't tolerate a baby aspirin. Aspirin may increase bruising in older people, but again, that's not very common.

I think the main reason people don't take aspirin is that their doctors don't tell them to. It's possible that doctors are just as concerned as everyone else about the risk of gastrointestinal irritation. If they haven't studied the issue, they may assume that aspirin can wreak havoc on a sensitive stomach. But they should know better, and they certainly should be familiar enough with the research to recognize that aspirin, even in very low doses, can be a lifesaving drug.

The Clot-Buster. So what, exactly, does aspirin do? Apart from its role as an analgesic, it reduces the ability of platelets to clump together or adhere to artery walls. Taking aspirin greatly reduces the odds that clots will form in the arteries; people who take it daily or every other day can reduce their risk of stroke and heart attack by 40% or more. The great thing about aspirin is that a single dose works for days. Once platelets lose their ability to clot, they stay out of commission for the rest of their cell-like lives. It's not until new platelets are formed in the bone marrow that the body's clotting mechanism returns to normal—at which point you just take another aspirin.

I should mention that aspirin does not prevent coronary artery disease. If you eat a high-fat diet, have high cholesterol, and neglect to exercise, you're going to develop fatty deposits that can potentially block the flow of blood to the heart. Aspirin doesn't stop this process. All it does is prevent clots. That's no small thing when you consider that heart attacks almost always occur when a clot jams one of the coronary arteries. If circulation isn't restored, the heart muscle will be permanently damaged, and you may or may not survive the experience.

One of the most important studies of recent years looked at 20,000 physicians over a period of five years. Half took aspirin daily, while the other half took a placebo. Researchers found that doctors who took aspirin were 44% less likely to get a first heart attack than those who didn't take aspirin. In doctors who already had heart disease, aspirin reduced their risk of a second heart attack by 33%, and their risk of stroke by 20%. These are truly remarkable benefits.

Unfortunately, all of the major studies to date have looked at aspirin's effects in men. We're pretty sure, but not positive, that it has the same effects in women. A large study looking at more than 44,000 nurses, which is currently in progress, should answer the question definitively. I expect that the results from this study will be available in the next three to five years.

Additional Benefits of Aspirin. Like the statins, aspirin's benefits go beyond protecting the heart. Everyone knows that aspirin is an excellent pain-reliever and anti-inflammatory. But one of the most intriguing findings of recent years is that aspirin appears to reduce the risk of colon cancer. Dartmouth University researchers recently reported that people who take a baby aspirin daily may reduce the formation of precancerous polyps in the colon by 19%. Taking aspirin in combination with statins—a good prescription for the millions of Americans at risk for heart disease—may reduce the risk of colon cancer by 20 to 30%.

Who Should Take Aspirin Daily? As is always the case with new treatments—or, in this case, old treatments with new uses—doctors can't agree who should be taking aspirin daily for preventive purposes. I recommend it to everyone over age 50, regardless of their overall health. There are only a few exceptions I can think of. If you're taking an anticoagulant such as warfarin, adding aspirin to the mix can increase your risk of internal bleeding. Similarly, some people have diseases that adversely affect the ability of platelets to function normally. Giving aspirin to someone with one of these conditions could cause out-of-control bleeding from the large intestine, or, in women, profuse bleeding during the menstrual period.

Also, some people are allergic to aspirin. My wife is one of them. If she takes even a single aspirin she develops angioneurotic edema, a condition that causes severe facial swelling. Aspirin allergies can also cause hives or a rapid heart rate. It's rare, but it does happen.

Assuming you aren't allergic to aspirin and your platelets are normal, do take it. The benefits far outweigh any possible risks. Don't let the fear of stomach upset put you off. It's true that some people are sensitive to even tiny amounts of aspirin. If you're one of them, take an enteric-coated preparation. Enteric-coated aspirin dissolves in the intestine rather than the stomach, which essentially eliminates the risk of stomach upset.

Dynamic Duo: ACE Inhibitors and Beta-Blockers

The drugs I've discussed so far are essential components in primary-prevention plans. If you have heart disease, or even if you don't, there's a good chance you should be taking aspirin and one of the statins. But what if your primary consideration is to prevent future problems after you've had a heart attack or been diagnosed with coronary artery disease? You almost certainly should be taking two additional drugs: an ACE inhibitor and a beta-blocker. Check your prescriptions: I'll bet even money that you're not getting them, and that's totally inexcusable.

ACE inhibitors and beta-blockers are among the most powerful drugs in our arsenals. If you have coronary artery disease or have had a heart attack, you absolutely have to take these drugs. If I sound a little passionate, it's because I have a personal interest. Six years ago, I had a mild heart attack, and it scared the hell out of me. I have no intention of going through it again, which is why I take lisinopril, an ACE inhibitor, and atenolol, a beta-blocker. (I also take aspirin and one of the statins, and I exercise regularly. There's nothing like a heart attack to jump-start your motivation.)

My advantage, of course, is that I can easily ferret out the latest medical literature, and I can also pick the brains of the cardiologists I work with. Most patients depend on the advice of their physicians, and that advice, I'm sad to say, isn't always the best. A while back, one of my patients came to see me after a visit to her cardiologist. She'd had a heart attack some years ago, and she also has kidney damage from diabetes. For whatever reason, her cardiologist didn't have her on ACE inhibitors or beta-blockers, which made no sense at all. A beta-blocker would significantly reduce her risk of a second heart attack. An ACE inhibitor would also protect her heart, while at the same time minimizing kidney damage from the diabetes. Fortunately, this lady is a voracious reader of health literature. She knows her stuff. After we talked, she went right back to her cardiologist and put the poor guy on the spot. She demanded to know why she wasn't getting the drugs. The cardiologist apologized for the oversight and wrote her a prescription on the spot. Love those assertive patients!

ACE Inhibitors. I can't stress it enough: These drugs are critical for those who have had heart attacks because they can prevent the subsequent development of heart failure. Drugs in this class, such as verapamil, captopril, Vasotec, Zestril, and Lotensin, block the formation of a hormone that indirectly triggers inflammation in damaged sections of coronary arteries. ACE inhibitors also help prevent the formation of life-threatening clots.

ACE inhibitors were originally developed to treat high blood pressure, but, as often happens with new drugs, their additional benefits soon became apparent. Research has clearly shown that these are among the most important drugs for those with heart disease or heart failure. And yet, doctors don't prescribe them anywhere near as much as they should. They may be so accustomed to using the drugs for high blood pressure that they're reluctant to give them to patients with heart conditions whose pressure is normal. There's also the misguided worry that the drugs will cause blood pressure to fall too low in those without hypertension. They do in fact cause a slight drop in systolic pressure in patients with normal blood pressure, but the drop is inconsequential.

As I mentioned earlier, one of the main uses of ACE inhibitors should be to prevent heart failure following a heart attack. Heart failure occurs when the heart weakens so much that it can't pump blood efficiently. Some of the main symptoms include shortness of breath, fluid retention, and sometimes an irregular heart beat. Heart failure is one of the main causes of death in the United States. The use of an ACE inhibitor reduces the risk of death from heart failure by 50%, and the need for repeated hospitalization by 60%. People who take these drugs following a heart attack are 21 to 37% less likely to die from severe heart failure than those who don't take them.

ACE inhibitors are also excellent drugs for the treatment of high blood pressure, the purpose for which they were first developed. They're not used routinely because other, cheaper drugs are generally just as effective. The exception is when high blood pressure is accompanied by diabetes, a combination that can severely damage the kidneys. ACE inhibitors appear to be particularly effective in preventing kidney damage in patients with diabetes. In more than 80% of cases, in fact, people who take these drugs have no further decline in kidney function. Anyone who has high blood pressure and kidney damage due to diabetes should be treated with an ACE inhibitor, unless there's a very good reason not to use the drugs.

Incidentally, there's some evidence that ACE inhibitors may prevent atherosclerosis, the buildup of fatty deposits in the arteries that is the main cause of heart attacks. Animal studies suggest that the drugs make cholesterol less likely to stick to artery walls and form the rigid coating, or plaque, that's the prime risk factor for blood clots. There's even some evidence that ACE inhibitors may reduce plaque deposits that have already formed. If these early findings turn out to apply to humans, then ACE inhibitors may eventually be used as much for preventing heart disease as treating it.

Cancer researchers have been looking at ACE inhibitors with new interest in recent years. The drugs appear to suppress inflammation and other changes in the body that can promote the development of cancer. Large studies have shown, in fact, that people with heart disease who take ACE inhibitors are about 30% less likely to get cancer than those who don't take the drugs.

The problem with most ACE inhibitors is they do cause significant side effects—serious drops in blood pressure, in some cases, or a severe cough. Fortunately, there's a new drug, Cozaar, which works in a similar fashion as ACE inhibitors, but which doesn't cause cough. It may be a better choice for some people.

Beta-Blockers. Beta-blockers get their name from the fact that they have a suppressing action on the beta-adrenergic system, a system largely controlled by the hormone noradrenaline. Noradrenaline increases heart rate and the strength of heart contractions. It constricts blood vessels and raises blood pressure. It also dilates the airways so you can pull in more air. The beta-adrenergic system is an important component of the fight-or-flight response—but in those with heart disease, all of this excitement can literally be overwhelming.

Beta-blockers essentially turn off the gas. Drugs in this class, such as propranolol, labetalol, carvedilol, and atenolol, slow the heart rate and lower blood pressure. They also decrease the force of the heart beat and help the heart relax between beats. This slowing action increases blood flow to the heart by reducing circulation to other parts of the body. They're absolutely wonderful drugs, and because they've been on the market for a long time, they're available in generic, inexpensive forms.

Nearly everyone who has had a heart attack *must* take a beta-blocker. They can reduce the risk of post–heart attack deaths by more than 40%. They can also prevent heart disease from progressing to heart failure. People who take beta-blockers have better cardiac function and fewer symptoms. They're less than half as likely to require hospital admission than heart failure patients who don't take the drugs. One study found that patients with heart failure who took a beta-blocker called carvedilol were 65% less likely to die from heart disease than similar patients who didn't get the drug. The benefits were so dramatic that the study was stopped three years early. Doctors felt it was unethical for any of the study participants to be given placebos when the benefits of the beta-blocker were so pronounced.

The drugs are useful in all age groups, but are particularly helpful in those 85 years and older. Studies have shown that elderly adults with heart disease who take beta-blockers can reduce their risk of death from heart disease by more than 20%.

The darned thing is, doctors tend not to use them. The only reason I can think of is that beta-blockers were once believed to worsen symptoms of heart failure. This has long since been disproved. If anything, beta-blockers generally help a failing heart. But old information dies hard. Only about 20% of people who should be taking beta-blockers are. Those who have had heart attacks need the drugs the most, yet less than 40% are taking them. Among patients with heart failure, only 30% or less are given beta-blockers.

Beta-blockers rarely cause serious complications, but they're not entirely safe, either. When you first start taking them, you have to begin with a low dose, which is gradually increased over time. Giving high doses too quickly can cause severe drops in blood pressure and cause the heart to slow too much. Blood pressure may drop precipitously, and, in rare cases, patients with heart failure do, in fact, get worse. In older people, the drugs may cause fatigue and depression. Many of these side effects can be avoided with proper dosing. And for the most part, the side effects of beta-blockers are mild and tend to disappear over time. One side effect that I worry about is depression. It mainly happens with the beta-blocker atenolol, which doesn't enter the brain as readily as other drugs. When this happens, switching to a different drug usually clears things up.

BE A PROACTIVE PATIENT

It always amazes me that in this era of physician shortages and cash-strapped hospitals, our health care system as a whole continues to favor invasive (and expensive) treatments for heart disease when medical management with medications is at least as effective, and a great deal cheaper. I suppose that taking action, any action, is emotionally more satisfying than merely writing a prescription. But whatever the reason, more than 50% of patients who should be getting drugs to reduce the risk of heart attacks, lower cholesterol, reduce arterial buildup, and prevent heart failure aren't getting them.

The appropriate use of drugs for treating heart problems is enormously complicated. Even specialists have a hard time keeping up with the latest findings. But this doesn't mean you have to passively accept whatever your doctor tells you. At the very least, please keep the following points in mind:

Insist on a statin drug if you have any risk factors for heart disease, including total cholesterol above 200 or LDL above 150. Statins are among the best ways to lower cholesterol and prevent heart attacks.

There's also good evidence that they protect against Alzheimer's disease and reduce the risk of some cancers.

Aspirin is truly a miracle drug. By the time you're 50, you should be taking it to reduce the risk of heart attack and stroke. Start with the lowest possible dose: 81.5 milligrams once a day. Your doctor may advise you to take slightly higher amounts for additional benefits.

If you've had a heart attack or have coronary artery disease or heart failure, treatment with both a beta-blocker and an ACE inhibitor is a must. The drugs reduce the risk of recurrent heart attacks and sudden death. They've also been shown to help prevent, and treat, heart failure.

If you already have coronary artery disease, plan on taking three drugs: aspirin, an ACE inhibitor, and a beta-blocker. Together, they provide tremendous benefits. Add a statin to the mix if your cholesterol is even slightly high.

The way we practice medicine isn't going to change overnight. I advise all of my patients to do everything they can, from reading textbooks to scouring the Internet, to become more knowledgeable about their health. When patients start pressing doctors to answer their questions—"How come you're not giving me a beta-blocker when such and such study proved it's effective?"— doctors will take it upon themselves to learn a little more.

CHAPTER SEVEN

*"I walk the dog every day. With my bad knees, that's about all
the exercise I can manage."*   *—Earl, age 68*

THE "SOFTENING"
OF EXERCISE ADVICE

I have a standard question that I ask whenever I meet with groups of
people. "If there were one thing that you could do that would
almost guarantee improved life expectancy and quality of life, and
that would reduce the risk of serious illnesses, would you do it?" The
answer—invariably, an overwhelming "Yes!"—is predictable.

Equally predictable is the groan that ripples through the room when
I say the word "exercise."

Perhaps 80% of Americans get little or no exercise. The health implications of our national sloth are enormous. Studies have shown, for
example, that someone who's obese but still exercises has a significantly
lower risk of heart disease and stroke than someone who looks to be in
good shape, but doesn't exercise. The trends of the last 20 years suggest
that it's the lack of exercise, rather than diet, that is responsible for the
36% increase in the numbers of those who are overweight. In the years
1980 to 1991—a time when the prevalence of obesity was surging—the
average calorie intake actually declined from 1850 to 1780 per day. At the

same time, total fat intake decreased by 11%. So the reason we're getting fat is *not* because we're eating more, but because we're not exercising.

It seems to me that the tendency to view exercise as a necessary evil has only increased in the wake of recent reports that suggest that people can get dramatic health gains with minimal exertion, such as walking at a snail's pace for half an hour a day—not even all at once, necessarily, but in "easy, 10-minute sessions." With that kind of advice floating around the scientific community and in the mainstream media, it's hardly surprising that people have hung up their tennis rackets and hauled the treadmill to a forgotten corner in the basement. Why get all tired and sweaty if a leisurely stroll around the block provides the same benefits?

But that's absolutely wrong-headed thinking. A leisurely stroll *won't* provide you the cardiac and strengthening benefits you need as you get older.

STROLLING WON'T DO IT

I'm not entirely sure how this "less is more" approach to exercise got started. So many studies have shown that people who are physically active stay healthier and live longer than those who are sedentary. Similarly, very modest amounts of exercise can promote weight loss and reduce the risk of diabetes and heart disease. This isn't surprising. We all know that some exercise is better than no exercise. But it hardly follows that some exercise is just as good as *more* exercise.

Consider a report that was recently published in the *New England Journal of Medicine*. The study showed that retired, nonsmoking men who walked regularly lived longer than those who didn't walk. The authors, quite correctly, pointed out the benefits of low-intensity physical activity. Yet there was more to the study than this. It also showed that men who walked less than a mile a day had twice the mortality rates of those who walked more than two miles. By any reasonable standards, a two-mile walk for someone aged 61 to 81 is a pretty hefty workout. But this part of the study didn't get a lot of attention. The media—and doctors—tended to focus more on the positive results gleaned from easy exercise, even though the benefits weren't anywhere near as pronounced as those provided by the tougher workouts.

Many of my patients, unfortunately, have taken these messages to heart. They're convinced that strolling a couple times a day will provide the same benefits as sweating through a really tough exercise session. The medical community, I'm afraid, is complicit in this unintentional ruse. Americans, on average, get so little exercise and are so out of shape that my colleagues and I are thrilled if we can get them to do anything more vigorous than walking to the refrigerator. A doctor who convinces a sedentary patient to commit to a walking program, even if it's only for half an hour three times a week, will feel a little glow of victory. But that much exercise, frankly, is nowhere near enough.

I recently suggested to my mom that she might want to set aside a little time for regular exercise. She looked at me and said, "Oy." That's a Yiddish word that roughly translates as, "How I suffer!" And the way she was looking at me when she said it, I know that I was the reason for all her grief and suffering. And here I was, suggesting that she exercise and suffer some more. "Oy, David, you are killing me. When I get the urge to exercise, I lie down and stay there until the urge goes away." I hear similar sentiments—minus the colorful language—from most of my patients.

I've given up trying to convince my mom to do anything, but I would like to convince you that the benefits of exercise are so varied, and so dramatic, that there's no rational excuse for not doing it. People who exercise have a much lower risk of diabetes, cancer, and heart disease.

Postmenopausal woman with mild hypertension who walk as little as 20 minutes daily can lower their systolic pressure into a healthful range. The same amount of exercise can reduce the risk of second heart attacks by 20%. People who exercise have stronger bones, better digestion, and healthier metabolisms. They're even less likely to get infections.

And remember, these benefits are from *minimal* amounts of exercise. When you exercise more, as everyone should, the benefits are much more pronounced.

THE PUSH-HARD PAYOFF

How much exercise do people really need? Is walking two miles a day enough for those 60 years and older? What about adults in their 40s and 50s?

I get asked these questions all the time, and my answer is always the same: Get more. If you currently exercise for 20 minutes at a time, increase it to 30 or 40 minutes. If you enjoy slow walking, pick up the pace and walk briskly. Increasing the time that you exercise, or exercising more intensely, will elevate what doctors call your exercise tolerance. The better your maximum exercise tolerance, the longer you're going to live.

A study of 13,485 Harvard alumni, with an average age of 58 years, compared the effects of light, moderate, and vigorous activity on longevity. Light activity, such as bowling, boating, and housekeeping, had no effect on life span. Moderate physical activity, which included golfing, dancing, and gardening, appeared to be somewhat beneficial. Those who exercised intensely, by running or swimming laps, for example, lived significantly longer.

The relationship between intense exercise and health is true for weight-lifting as well as aerobic types of exercise. I wish more of my patients lifted weights because it provides astonishing health benefits. Weight lifting, also called resistance training, increases strength, improves gait and balance, and reduces age-related bone loss. It also lowers the risk of diabetes because muscle tissue takes up glucose, or blood sugar, much more readily than fat tissue. I'll talk about weight lifting in more detail later, but for now I'll just repeat the one message that we all need to hear: More is almost always better.

In the last 20 years or so, physical trainers and physiologists have made a point of debunking the weight lifter's traditional mantra, "No pain, no gain." It's certainly true that exercising to the point of pain and beyond can damage muscles or joints. People who push themselves too hard, without adequate preparation, are more likely to get hurt than fit. It's also true that you can achieve some health and fitness gains with a laid-back, no-sweat style of lifting. But when I see people casually lifting free weights or working out on exercise machines, I want to shout, "Push harder!" There's simply no substitute for hard effort. Research has clearly shown that for weight lifting to have a significant effect on muscles and bones, you have to strain. Sorry, but it's true. If you hardly feel anything after lifting a weight ten times, you're not working anywhere near hard enough.

AGING MUSCLES AND BONES

An unfortunate fact of aging is that muscle mass and strength inexorably decline after you've reached your late 20s or early 30s. By age 50, muscle mass is about 70% of what it was at age 30. By the time people reach their 80th birthday they will have lost more than 50% of their peak muscle mass. Sad to say, overall body weight stays about the same because the loss of muscle is usually accompanied by an increase in fat. Even if your weight has remained constant over the decades, you'll have proportionately more fat at age 55 than you did at 25.

Muscle Loss

What causes this gradual reduction in muscle and the concomitant increase in fat? A lack of exercise certainly is one reason, but it's not the only one. There appear to be biological changes that result in age-related muscle loss. We're recently discovered that primitive muscle cells called myoblasts proliferate as muscle fibers diminish. Myoblasts mature into cells called myocytes, which repair damaged muscles and replace muscle fibers that have been destroyed by injuries.

The ability of myocytes to repair muscle appears to diminish over time. In addition, there's some evidence that an older person's myoblasts, rather than maturing into muscle-building myocytes, get "diverted" and form more fat cells. These effects are in full swing by age 50, and they continue with advancing age.

We're still not sure what reduces the ability of myocytes to function normally. Genetic changes might be involved. It could also be due to decades of exposure to oxidants—byproducts of metabolism that damage cells throughout the body. As we learn more about the things that damage myocytes, we may someday be able to manipulate the genetic composition of myoblasts, make them young again, and perhaps prevent age-related muscle declines. But this is a long way in the future. For now, the only way to build muscle tissue is with exercise—and the older you get, the more important it becomes.

Bone Loss

The progressive loss of muscle, if it isn't reversed with exercise, has profound implications. For example, muscle weakness is a direct cause of the age-related bone loss, or osteoporosis, that affects millions of older adults. Men can and do get osteoporosis, but it's more common in women. Bone loss accelerates for several years after women reach menopause, and then it slows somewhat. But it never stops entirely. The bones often get so weak that they spontaneously fracture. Even if the bones hold together, osteoporosis is a major cause of aches and pains, as well as significant disability.

The combination of muscle weakness and thin bones is a prescription for disaster. Falls resulting in fractures are one of the most common causes of dependency in older adults, as well as a leading cause of death. More than half of those 75 years and older who break a hip will never walk normally again. Many, in fact, are admitted to nursing homes, where they often die within one year. What drives me crazy is that the vast majority of these complications could be prevented if only people would commit to vigorous exercise.

All of us tend to get more sedentary as we get older. Muscles that aren't worked get progressively weaker, which reduces their ability to maintain the integrity of joints. Combined with normal wear and tear on the joints, this can lead to osteoarthritis, the most common chronic medical problem after age 50. Joint pain is often the reason we stop running, playing tennis, or even walking. Thus begins a terrible cycle. Unused muscles keep getting weaker. Weak muscles fail to support the joints. The joints get increasingly stiff and painful, and so we exercise even less.

Here's another reason that exercise is so important for older adults. If you're sedentary, you have a greater proportion of fat and a smaller proportion of muscle. Unlike muscle tissue, which requires a lot of calories to function normally, fat is relatively inert. It requires very little in the way of subsistence, which means that you naturally take in fewer calories. That might sound like a good thing, but keep in mind that your need for protein and other nutrients doesn't decline. If anything, it increases. But if you have a diminished need for calories, how will you get enough nutrients? The short answer is that you won't. About half of those 70 years and older get insufficient amounts of protein, calcium, iron, and other essential vitamins and minerals. Here in the affluent United States, malnutrition and even starvation are facts of life among hospitalized or ill elderly adults.

The gradual accumulation of fat, and the loss of muscle tissue, is dangerous in yet another way. These changes reduce the ability of insulin—the hormone that carries glucose (blood sugar) into the body's cells—to function normally. This condition, called insulin resistance, can lead to or worsen diabetes, the devastating disease that vastly increases the risk for heart disease, stroke, blindness, and nerve disorders.

We cannot stop the loss of muscle that occurs with aging. Nor is it possible to turn 80-year-old bones into the bones of a teenage athlete. What we can do is make the bones much stronger, and prevent virtually all of the negative effects just by exercising. I cannot emphasize this enough. We, the baby boomers, are approaching the time in our lives when the risks of physical disability and dependence are rising. Our parents are already there. We'd be crazy not to do something about it.

Exercise Won't Hurt You!

Well, maybe we are crazy. Among my patients, there's a general attitude that hard exercise is best left to the younger folks. This is partly due, I'm sure, to our lifelong patterns of excuses for not exercising. But I think that there's some fear involved. When your energy isn't what it used to be, or your knees hurt or your back feels weak, or you're seeing a doctor for chronic health problems, the idea of vigorous exercise is a little scary.

What if you break something? What if your body simply can't handle the strain?

Let me put this to rest. There's absolutely no increase in illness or great risk of injury when people 70 years and older engage in strenuous aerobic or resistance exercises. Quite the contrary. Older adults stand to gain even more from vigorous exercise than younger folks.

A walking program by itself can modestly improve bone strength. Add weight lifting to the mix, and there will be a dramatic improvement in spine and femur (leg bone) strength. Hard exercise in older adults significantly improves posture, gait, and balance. Studies suggest that high-intensity weight training can reduce the risk of falls by 80%. Evidence is also emerging that vigorous exercise improves mental abilities, probably because it increases blood flow to the brain.

An intriguing study examined the benefits of high-intensity resistance training in nursing home patients over the age of 90. The results were astounding. After eight weeks of high-intensity training, people in the study had strength increases of 174%. Yes, you read that right: *174%*. Muscle mass increased more than 10%, and their walking speed shot up by 48%.

Based on this and other research, my advice is simple: Do as much as you can, then find in yourself the motivation to do more. If you exercised vigorously at age 30—or 40, 50, or 60—keep it up. If, on the other hand, you were never all that physically active, now's the time to start. It doesn't matter if all you can do is walk up and down the stairs. Make the climb—and throw in a few minutes of extra walking. When you work in the yard, move more quickly than usual. Push yourself. I know, exercise doesn't feel very good at first. You're going to tire quickly, and you might be a little sore. But if you push yourself just a little harder, your strength and endurance will increase faster than you can imagine.

Fortunately, a significant segment of the population is now hooked on exercise. No matter where I go, I see crowds of proud and healthy joggers, hikers, and walkers. The age of new members at health clubs is getting progressively older. Silver hair and wrinkles, rather than twenty-something radiance, may well become the rule rather than the exception. I hope so.

EXERCISE EXCUSES

Researchers have spent a lot of time investigating why so few of us exercise. Why is it that an activity that is so manifestly beneficial is viewed with so much disdain? First, there are genetic and physiological factors. Some people may be genetically predisposed to have good flexibility, balance, and strength, all qualities that obviously make exercise feel more natural. It's a lot easier for the "natural athletes" among us to maintain physically active lifestyles than it is for those who have always had limited endurance or been somewhat clumsy. Everyone can develop reasonable levels of strength and endurance, but the effort will be harder for those who have been sedentary most of their lives.

Honestly, it takes a lot of motivation to begin and stick with any new exercise plan. Unfortunately, it often seems to take a catastrophic event, like a heart attack, to provide the wake-up call. Even then, motivation can be fleeting. People who have recently been diagnosed with heart disease usually make all sorts of resolutions—to go to the gym every day, to wake up earlier to get in a morning walk, and so on. As the months go by, however, complacency often returns and they drift back to their old, slothful ways.

People always have reasons why getting regular exercise is flat-out impossible. I've found that these reasons usually involve the word "too."

I am too busy, too tired, too sick, too old, too weak, too fat, or too intimidated. Let's take a look at the most common exercise excuses—and see how lame they really are!

I'm too busy. This one never holds up very well. Nearly everyone can get a thoroughly vigorous workout in 20 to 30 minutes. If you're really so busy that you can't set aside half an hour a day, than your priorities need adjusting. Get up half an hour earlier in the morning. Give up the evening news. Forget the afternoon nap. Whatever it takes, set aside the time to exercise. People who are truly so busy that they can't find time to exercise are looking at a grim future.

In my experience, people who say they're too busy to exercise are really saying that they're too stressed. That by itself is going to lead to illness. Combined with a lack of exercise, stress is one of the major killers because it significantly increases the risk for high blood pressure, heart disease, and cancer. The darned thing is, it's so easy to reverse. If you exercise you'll have less stress. You'll feel better, function better, and enjoy life more. Simple as that. And ultimately, you'll find that you have more time than you thought because exercise boosts energy and productivity.

I'm too tired. Fatigue is usually caused by stress, poor sleep, depression, the use of some medications, or illness. Don't ignore fatigue, especially if it's so pronounced that you feel you can't exercise because of it. Talk to your doctor and come up with a solution. Chances are, there's nothing seriously wrong with you, and you just have to get started. One of the best ways to treat fatigue is to exercise. It improves metabolism and promotes better sleep. It also stimulates the release of hormones and cytokines, natural chemicals that promote feelings of energy and well-being.

I'm too sick. Obviously, I wouldn't advise anyone with a bad cold to jog three miles on an icy morning. But what if you have a long-term illness—severe arthritis, for example, or cancer or heart disease? The evidence is compelling that exercise is important in the recovery of every major disease. A study of patients with osteoarthritis, for example, showed that intensive exercise—both aerobic and resistance training—significantly reduced symptoms and disability. Exercise is also an integral part of rehabilitation following a heart attack or open heart surgery. In fact, people who take up an exercise program are three times less likely to have further heart problems.

And let's not forget the preventive aspects of exercise. Studies have shown that people who are physically active have about half the colon cancer risk as those who are sedentary. Evidence also suggests that exercise reduces the risk of breast and prostate cancers by modulating hormone levels.

I'm too old. Forget it. I'm not buying that one. The evidence is very clear that older adults who exercise feel better, live longer, and have fewer physical problems. As I mentioned earlier, even nursing home patients—who, by definition, are the frailest of the frail—can have threefold improvements in strength when they lift weights. Their balance gets better and they're much less likely to fall and be injured. In fact, just about every measure of health improves.

The ability to exercise does decline with age, of course. You won't be as strong at 70 as you were at 20, and you won't have quite as much endurance. That doesn't matter at all. As long as you're always pushing yourself a little harder and farther, you're going to benefit. Think about those magnificent people who, at age 70 and beyond, compete in—and complete—the New York Marathon!

I'm in too much pain. It is true that pain may limit your ability to exercise, and you don't want to exercise right after an injury. But chronic pain, such as that caused by arthritis, is not a reason to quit exercising.

It may change the kind of exercise undertaken, but not the ability to exercise. Studies have clearly shown that a cornerstone of therapy for back pain involves physical activity, supervised exercises, and stretching. The same is true of arthritis. More exercise invariably means less pain.

I'm too fat and I look lousy in tights. I can't say I blame anyone who's reluctant to exercise where anyone can see them. I feel this way myself. Who wants to go to a gym or a running trail and be surrounded by impossibly fit people with tiny waists and imposing muscles? It may be helpful to remind yourself that you're probably paying more attention to them than they are to you. I've talked to a lot of these "beautiful" people, and they always say that the last things they're thinking about, let alone noticing, are the body shapes or fitness levels of their less-in-shape counterparts. Believe me, they probably won't even know you're there. Or, if they do, they're probably having the opposite perception of what you might think. Rather than judging you critically, they're probably admiring your initiative and spunk.

One of my friends, a 25-year-old woman, once told me, "The three older women who work out together at my gym amaze me. They're well into their sixties and they're there more often than I am. I'm not thinking about how they have more wrinkles than me. I'm thinking, my gosh, I want to be that dedicated and active when I'm that old."

I hate to exercise. I hate to say it, but this one's hard to argue with. Some people don't like doing crossword puzzles, some don't like bowling, and others, I'm afraid, don't like to exercise. All I can say is, get over it. I doubt you like flossing your teeth, but you do it anyway. You might not like exercise, but I guarantee you, you'll like having a heart attack a lot less.

Actually, I doubt very much that there's anyone in the world who truly dislikes all forms of physical activity. When people say they hate to exercise, what they usually mean is that they hate some of the activities they've tried in the past. Me, I dislike jogging with a passion. It took me awhile to discover how much I like riding a stationary bike. You'll surely find an exercise that's right for you. It could be biking, swimming, tennis, or walking the dog. If you make the commitment that you're going to exercise *no matter what*, you'll eventually find something that agrees with you.

Besides, I've found that it's not exercise, per se, that puts people off, but other factors, like being out of shape or feeling tired or stressed. Once they start exercising, and they realize how much better they feel afterward, they generally come around.

So far, I've been talking about exercise in the most general terms. All forms of exercise are so beneficial that it doesn't matter all that much what kinds you do. But if you want to get the most benefits—cardio-vascular fitness along with gains in strength, balance, and mobility—you'll have to combine aerobic and strength-training exercises.

THE AEROBIC EDGE

Let's start with aerobic exercise, which simply means any activity that increases your heart and respiratory rates. Strictly speaking, getting up from a chair is aerobic exercise. For real health and fitness gains, of course, aerobic exercise has to give the heart and lungs a tough workout. Whether you're swimming, jogging, biking, dancing, or walking, the ideal goal is to elevate your heart rate to between 60 and 80% of its top rate.

Don't get thrown by the numbers. This is an easy calculation to make. First, subtract your age from 220. If you're 55 years old, for example, your top heart rate is somewhere around 165 beats a minute. A good aerobic workout will raise your heart rate to 60 to 80% of that. In this case, that's between 99 and 132 beats a minute. Plan on maintaining that heart rate for at least 30 minutes, and get the exercise at least three to five days a week.

It's impossible to summarize the benefits of aerobic exercise in just a few words, but here are the main ones.

A stronger heart. After each heartbeat, the heart relaxes and fills with blood prior to the next contraction that forces the blood out. This relaxation period is called diastole. Many older Americans develop a condition called diastolic dysfunction, which means the heart doesn't relax sufficiently to admit enough blood, especially during exertion. This can cause breathlessness, weakness, and, eventually, heart failure. Regular aerobic exercise can prevent this unpleasant sequence of events.

Improved heart function. Everyone who's middle-aged or older has some degree of cholesterol depositions in the heart and arteries. Even in those without symptoms, the blockage can be quite extensive, and it does get worse with age. Aerobic exercise can help prevent heart attacks by improving blood flow to the heart. It also improves the ability of the heart to contract forcefully as well as to relax. This improves heart function, reduces the risk of heart failure and high blood pressure, and helps you live longer.

Good exercise for the lungs. Since aerobic exercise makes you breathe faster, it's excellent exercise for the lungs. It helps remove mucus from the airways and can even minimize damage caused by smoking or air pollution.

Enhanced mood. Study after study has shown that aerobic exercise can improve mood, reduce the risk of depression, and increase energy and work performance. By any objective (and subjective) measure, it improves the quality of life.

The most important part of aerobic exercise is choosing something you enjoy. Jogging, swimming, walking, treadmills, and exercise bikes are all good choices—but not necessarily for you. Exercise is a real chore unless it's something that you enjoy so much that you'd do it even if it weren't good for you.

RESISTANCE TRAINING

People tend to think of weight lifting as a hobby for the young and fit, but it's a lot more than that. I can't think of a single lifestyle change that's more beneficial than lifting weights at least a few times a week. If you were to use a CT scan to look at two thighs, one belonging to a 20-year-old and the other to someone in their 80s, you'd see a remarkable difference. The thigh of a 20-year-old is about 80% muscle; in the older adult, it's mainly fat.

Weight lifting can dramatically increase muscle size and strength in people of all ages. What's most intriguing is that the benefits of weight training increase as we get older. Earlier, I mentioned new research that found that nursing home residents who participated in a weight-training program were able to triple their muscle size and strength, while at the same time dramatically reducing their risk of falls. These points are worth emphasizing because fall-induced fractures in the United States are incredibly common, and cost $80 billion annually.

Weight training has become an integral part of the rehabilitation of older adults who can't get around on their own. Improvements in strength and balance aren't the only reasons. Lifting weights builds larger muscles. Muscle is metabolically more active than fat, which means that people who do weight training have increased appetite and tend to gain weight. This might not be an important goal for younger people, but it's critical in the elderly, who frequently are underweight and may not get all the nutrients that they need to be healthy. As far as we know, only a combination of resistance training and an adequate diet has these effects. Without exercise, appetite does not improve and food intake stays constant. Even dietary supplements, such as milkshakes or prepared formulas, won't do a thing for appetite unless exercise is included in the program.

On the few occasions I've been to the gym, I notice that a lot of people, young and old alike, tend to lift weights that don't appear to challenge them very much. I hate to say it, but just lifting a small dumbbell, one that hardly taxes your reserves, isn't worth the effort. Every study that has shown substantial benefits from resistance training involved high-intensity, muscle-taxing exercises.

In practical terms, this means choosing weights that are sufficiently heavy that the muscle is virtually exhausted after six to eight repetitions of the exercise. According to exercise physiologists, you'll get the most benefits when the muscles are "exercised to 80% of a single maximum repetition." Suppose that you choose a weight that's so heavy that you can only lift it once. Obviously, that's too heavy to get much of a workout. You want to start out by lifting 80% of that amount, and repeating the exercise six to eight times. When you can complete the exercise eight times without being totally exhausted, it's time to increase the weight.

Sound like hard work? It is, believe me. But it's the only way to build your strength to the level it needs to be for optimal fitness. You'll probably be a little sore when you first start out. The soreness goes away pretty quickly, and you'll find that you feel refreshed and energized after your workouts. Your muscles will be tired, but they won't hurt.

Weight training should be done under the supervision of a trainer or physical therapist, at least until you learn the ropes. Unlike walking or biking, which are almost impossible to do wrong, weight training requires proper form and technique. Barbells, dumbbells, and other kinds of "free" weights provide a superb workout, but they do require more balance—and, in many cases, strength—than machine weights. Some health clubs have started using elastic bands instead of weights. Different bands provide different levels of resistance, and they may be less daunting to beginners than clanking iron bars and plates.

I don't recommend the use of home equipment. Apart from the initial expense, it's hard to stay motivated when your workout room is a musty corner of the basement. Health clubs are a much better choice. There are people on staff who can explain how to use the weights properly and reduce the risk of getting hurt. Health clubs are also a lot of fun because it's a way to get out of the house and meet new people. Don't worry, you won't be the only beginner, and you certainly won't be the only adult over age 30. Those perfect (and intimidating) bodies are the exception, not the rule. Whether you've been active all your life or are just starting out, you and your physique will feel right at home.

GETTING STARTED

When I was in my early 30s, jogging was the craze. Like many of my friends, I decided to take it up. I can't say that I ever enjoyed it, but four times a week for five years, I religiously pounded the pavements. I jogged about three miles a day, and I can still see myself, a lumbering elephant, struggling up those mild inclines with a frown on my face. I won't dwell on the shin splints, joint pains, and occasional twilight tumbles in the dark that plagued my foray into fitness. Suffice it to say that this was probably the worst form of exercise for me. After awhile, I found myself coming up with all sorts of excuses for skipping my runs. Finally, I pretty much stopped altogether. And gained more weight than I care to admit.

At the time, I had all sorts of explanations why exercise wasn't working for me. Then, a few years ago, I got the inevitable wake-up call. A day after returning from a 32-hour flight from Malaysia, I went to visit a terminally ill patient at home. I'd planned to help him die in comfort, but instead I developed rather severe chest pain—a mild heart attack, I discovered soon enough.

From that day on, my commitment to improve my health never faltered again. I became a prime example of my often-repeated mantra: "It's never too early, or too late, to start exercising." I knew that jogging wasn't going to work for me. I tried a treadmill, and that didn't work either. That's when I discovered the joy of indoor bikes. I watch TV while I pedal away, and the time pretty much flashes by. I also discovered the pleasures of brisk walking, which raises my heart rate to an adequate level without making my bones and joints ache.

It took a long time, but I finally found my own little exercise niche. Today, I alternate indoor biking with one-hour walks. I also resistance-train two to three times weekly, and I've never felt better.

See your doctor first. I do advise people who haven't exercised before, or those who are elderly and may have other health problems, to see their doctor before lacing up their athletic shoes. You want to be sure that you aren't at risk for a sudden heart attack or other health problems when you put your body under more strain than it's accustomed to. If you're really out of shape, you might need to overcome the effects of deconditioning—a fancy way of saying that you have so little muscle and stamina that even mild exercise leaves you exhausted, breathless, and weak. You may need to work with a physical therapist, who will put you on a program of graded exercise, in which you very gradually build up your endurance.

Recruit a friend. If you've been sedentary for a lot of years, you're going to have a couple of difficult weeks when you first start exercising. Your body won't be used to moving, and it's going to let you know. Your mind is going to rebel, as well. Until exercise becomes a habit, which it will within about a month, you're going to have to depend on willpower to make it happen. You might want to find a fellow soul-mate and arrange times to get together. It's a lot easier to stick with the plan when someone else is around to keep you company—and to give you a kick in the behind when you start making excuses!

Keep at it. Even though 30 minutes or more of aerobic exercise is ideal, you should think of this as a target to aim for, rather than something to achieve immediately. If you've been sedentary for a long time, plan on doing some brisk aerobic exercise for five to 10 minutes. If you're breathless, you're pushing too hard and will need to back off. Don't get discouraged. Just keep at it. Your tolerance for exercise will improve very quickly. You'll probably be hitting the 30-minute target within a month or two, and possibly sooner.

Aim high. Even though I advise everyone to begin with a few baby steps, you do want to set your expectations high. Each and every one of us has a mountain that we can climb. For some, the peak is as high as the Himalayas. For others, it's the height of a curb. But as long as you take those first steps, you'll see amazing progress.

JUST DO IT!

I can't stress enough that exercise is the key to continued good health. Americans are getting less and less fit because we tend to focus almost exclusively on diet, and even when exercise enters the equation, the fitness prescriptions are unrealistically low. If you're already active, keep it up! Know that you're dramatically improving your chances of a longer, happier, more independent life. For those of you who have never exercised, I hope that this chapter has given you the inspiration to start. You can do it—and believe me when I tell you that it really is worth it.

CHAPTER EIGHT

*"No, we don't make love anymore. But that's okay. I don't
miss it, not really. We have a good time—we go out to dinner
with friends, play cards, watch movies together. I'm too old for
sex now. I don't think Sam cares, either."* —Barbara, age 63

"Doc, any chance I could get a sample of Viagra from you?"
—Sam, age 66

HAVE MORE SEX!
YOU'LL LIVE LONGER!

Is it nature's plan for our sexual futures to go inexorably downhill?
When we're 60, 70, or 80, are we condemned to struggle with infrequent or unsatisfying sex? Research suggests that the answer is no.
The reason so many older couples and singles have little or no sex has
more to do with outlook and imagination than with sexual machinery.
True, we all slow down. Both men and women tend to require more time
and stimulation as they get older.

But I see no drawbacks in this. The evidence is clear that older adults,
as a group, often have better sex than they did when they were younger.
And they certainly have more and better sex than the popular clichés—
desperate dowagers, impotent codgers—would have you believe.

Satisfaction aside, there are good medical reasons to cultivate all the passion you can handle. People who maintain good relationships and active sex lives stay healthier and live longer than those without this spice.

I had an interesting discussion with a colleague while I was working on this chapter a few days ago. He said that after 25 years of marriage, he had come to the conclusion that he was madly in love with his wife, totally and without reservation. Their relationship was hardly without problems. They had the usual conflicts, mainly about money (there was always too little) and sex (there was never enough). But over the years, they fought less and appreciated each other more. And in most ways, he said, the sex had never been better. Maybe not as frequent as it once was, but sexier and more passionate. And as a result, my colleague and his wife, with 25 years of marriage behind them, are statistically likely to have long, fulfilling lives.

Many of us, sad to say, aren't so lucky in our relationships. It's easy to see my friend's happy story as an exception to the hard realities of many long-term marriages. I must tell another story to illustrate this point. I grew up in South Africa and emigrated to the United States in the early 1970s, when the problems of apartheid became unbearable. I still talk to some of my childhood friends, but my mother, social butterfly that she is, keeps in touch with all of them. She doesn't hesitate to use this inside information to let me know just how much I've disappointed her.

At least once a year, she puts her hand on my arm and says, "Do you remember Howard?" She knows very well that I do. Howard was one of my childhood friends. I've known him, in fact, since we were in kindergarten. "He's done very well," she goes on. "He's the CEO of a large company in Sacramento. He's made a fortune!"

The last time we had this conversation, I'd actually run into Howard a few months before. From what I could tell, he hadn't done very well at all. His business was certainly successful, but his life was a mess. His first wife divorced him because he was quick to anger, was rarely at home, and neglected their three beautiful children. His second wife came and went before I got a chance to meet her. When Howard and I ran into each other, he was with his current fiancée, young enough to be his daughter.

"You call this jerk successful?" I thought to myself. He smokes, never exercises, and is overweight. The pressures of a falling stock market may do him in. And he confided, when we were alone, that the Prozac he was taking for depression had "shot my sex life to hell." Before we said goodbye, he asked if I would write him a prescription for Viagra.

Every year, it seems, more and more of my friends and acquaintances—and a great many of my patients—have followed a similar path, at least in terms of their relationships. Many of the couples I've known for years are getting divorced. They're unhappy and lonely. They dip in and out of relationships, but nothing really seems to click. The sex that once seemed so natural is fraught with difficulties. The men struggle with erection problems. The women have fewer orgasms or have trouble with lubrication. All in all, they seem trapped in a dismal sexual cycle, with poor body images, an utter lack of spice and excitement, and the painful yearning for younger, more virile days.

SEX IS FOREVER

I suspect that we all look back somewhat wistfully at our younger, presumably more sexual, selves. But when we take an honest look through the pleasant haze of memory, most of us would agree that our early sex lives weren't all that great. For women, especially, worries about pregnancy can take a lot of the steam out of sex. There are endless distractions: job or money worries, crying babies, kids coming home from school. Inexperience is its own kind of cold shower. I don't know about you, but I was much more nervous about sex in my younger years than I am today. I worried about pleasing my partner. I was often too embarrassed to say what I liked or didn't like, or to frankly ask my partners what they liked. Sex tended to feel like a performance—one with a potentially harsh judge! It wasn't until I was much older and more confident that sex become more about sharing pleasures and less about proving something about myself.

Sex Gets Better with Age

Our attitudes toward sex do change with age. And there's no escaping the fact that our bodies change. If you expect to function exactly the same at 80 as you did at 20, get ready for disappointment. But most of us, I think, know better than to confuse stamina or vigor with sexual satisfaction. I'm certainly less of an athlete than I was 30 years ago, but the pleasure that I get from sex has increased beyond measure.

So much of the popular information about the effects of aging on sex is either misleading or flat-out wrong. Every major scientific study that I'm aware of shows that the interest in and need for sex does not decrease with age. Research has shown, for example, that 60% of men and women ages 45 to 59 have sex at least once weekly. As they get older, the frequency of sex diminishes, but it never tapers off completely. About 87% of married men and 89% of married women ages 60 to 64 remain sexually active. In those 75 years and older, about 25% have intercourse at least once a week.

Older couples may have sex less often, but they enjoy it every bit as much. Most couples (to the horror of their children) remain sexually active throughout their lives. Should they suddenly lose their partners to death or divorce, they miss the sex a great deal. Just recently, a friend told me how shocked she was when her grandmother, a woman of 80, confessed that she didn't miss her late husband at all, but she sure missed the sex!

An interesting thing happens in older age groups. After age 75, men start having more sex than women. Specifically, about 58% of men 75 years and older continue to have sex, while only 25% of women do. Does this mean that women lose their interest in sex? Not at all. Women live longer than men, and in these older age groups, there are simply too few men to go around. So the men who are still energetic and healthy are having more sex, while women have to make do with less.

I realize that my conviction that sex gets better with age—a message that I fervently stress to my patients—is something of a hard sell. We're inundated with media messages that tell us that "sexy" and "young" are synonymous, that if you have gray hair, wrinkles, and a less-than-perfect body, sex is probably unattainable, certainly unsatisfying, and possibly a little unappetizing. But the vast amount of sexuality research that has been conducted in the last few decades, along with the zesty stories I hear from my less-inhibited patients, suggest something quite different. Yes, sex changes. It might change for the worse in some people—those with serious health problems, for example, or those who were never all that interested in (or comfortable with) the sexual sides of themselves. But for many others, sex gets, well, sexier, with advancing age.

Let me share some intriguing statistics. Between the ages of 18 and 31, for example, only about 23% of men and 31% of women report being "very happy" with their sex lives. In those over age 65, on the other hand, the percentage jumps to 48. The National Council on Aging conducted a survey of more than 1200 older adults. The survey found that 50% of men and women aged 60 and older remained sexually active, and about 70% of them were happier with their sex lives than they had been in their 40s.

Dr. Patricia Bloom, a leading sexuality expert, has a number of theories as to why sex seems to get more satisfying with advancing years. Her research suggests that older adults, with their years of experience, develop a sense of freedom and confidence that they didn't have when they were younger. In other words, they often shed many of their inhibitions. They aren't shy about masturbating. They're willing to experiment and find new ways of getting pleasure, either with new or lifelong partners. It's not uncommon for elderly women to redefine their entire sexual universe by developing relationships with same-sex partners, even when they spent most of their lives in heterosexual relationships. Clearly, sexual adventure and experimentation aren't the prerogatives of youth. Quite the opposite. Older adults are *more* likely to define and express their sexuality in more varied ways.

MORE SEX, A LONGER LIFE

It makes intuitive sense that good sex, however you define "good," improves the quality of life. That alone is sufficient reason for everyone, at all stages of life, to stay sexually active. But forget the feel-good aspects of sex for a moment. There's also a strong correlation between sexual activity and longevity.

A study reported in the *British Medical Journal* found that men who had frequent orgasms—more than two a week—were 50% less likely to die in a given period than those who had orgasms less than once a month. Men who had sex twice a week were three times less likely to have a heart attack than those who had sex less than once a month.

Other studies have arrived at similar conclusions. I wish I could explain why sex appears to be protective, but the research is a little murky. We know that married men live longer than those who are single, widowed, or divorced, and they also have sex more frequently. It's possible that marriage, rather than sex, is what caused these men to do better. Or maybe sex stimulates physical changes in the body that promote long-term health. For now, we just don't know.

Incidentally, what's good for the gander appears to be equally beneficial for the goose—but with a twist. While sexual frequency is directly linked to longevity in men, sexual satisfaction is much more important for women. Researchers at Duke University's Center on Aging have found that the enjoyment of sex is a powerful predictor of reduced mortality. In other words, women who enjoy sex live longer, regardless of how often they have it. Conversely, women who are dissatisfied with their sex lives are more likely to have heart attacks than those who are sexually satisfied.

There's really no question that sex is good for your health, and the more sex you have, the healthier you're likely to be. But good sex, as we all know, doesn't exist in isolation. No matter how turned on you get when you look at attractive people, read suggestive material, or watch erotic movies, you're going to get the most satisfaction, and excitement, when you're having sex with someone you love. This sounds downright old-fashioned, but it's true: People in committed relationships have more sex than those "swinging" singles, and they rate their overall sexual satisfaction a lot higher. Studies have shown, for example, that sexual satisfaction is about 20% higher for married couples than for those who have lived together for a year or more.

This satisfaction apparently translates to good health. In Canada, Europe, and the United States, married men live an average of eight years longer than men who have never been married, and 10 years longer than widowers. Married women don't benefit as much, but benefit they do. Women who are married live about three years longer than women who have never married, and four years longer than those who have been divorced or widowed. Studies have shown, in fact, that married men and women have lower risks of heart disease and cancer. It's possible that having a caring and supportive partner improves overall coping skills. Emotional support clearly reduces stress, which has been linked to dozens of chronic and life-threatening illnesses. People who are in committed relationships are also more likely to pay attention to their health—by exercising and eating nutritious meals, for example— than those who go it alone.

Let's look at some of the other health benefits of being in a stable relationship. Married couples have lower rates of depression and alcohol and substance abuse. People who are married are less likely to commit suicide, probably because they feel more connected and less lonely. Studies have shown, for example, that 30% of those who have been separated report feeling lonely, compared to only 4% of married couples.

While I was researching this chapter, I read just about every book on the subject, along with dozens of scientific reports. What struck me most was that the benefits of being in a long-term, committed relationship appeared in just about every aspect of life. For example, a large survey conducted in 1998 found that older married couples were more likely to exercise than their single counterparts. They were more likely to wear seat belts. They got their blood pressure checked regularly. They were less likely to drink or smoke. They were even more likely to eat breakfast.

For most of the measures, men who were married benefited somewhat more than the women. This doesn't surprise me. In my experience, it almost takes a crowbar to get an older man into a doctor's office, and nothing short of a force of nature will commit them to making healthful lifestyle changes. Women take their health more seriously, and they are rarely shy about pushing their husbands in the same direction. For older men, regular badgering by a concerned wife is one of the most under-recognized facets of good health care.

I don't think many people would disagree that it's this intimacy and connectedness—even the loving badgering—that makes for great sex. Men and women see things somewhat differently, of course. Women tend to demand intimacy, touching, and communication. Men tend to focus more on the act itself. Men, we have to do better! The only way we can reap the benefits of long-term relationships—more exciting sex, better health, and a longer life—is to approach sex more as women do. Be considerate, caring, understanding. Where there's intimacy, there's good sex. And with good sex comes a happier—and longer—life.

SEX AND THE CHANGING BODY

It's worth taking a moment to discuss some of the physical changes that we all experience as we get older. But please remember: There's no reason for these natural, age-related changes to dampen ardor or inhibit good love-making. You might have to make some adjustments—allowing more time to get aroused, for example, or taking advantage of modern pharmaceuticals—but that's hardly unique to sex. I'd love to give up my glasses or wake up in the morning as limber as a teenager. Since I can't, I make the necessary accommodations.

Changes in Men

For men, the height of sexual functioning occurs at about age 18. Young men can often have multiple erections and orgasms on any given night, and they can repeat the performance night after night. The irony, of course, is that men of this age are unlikely to have steady relationships or the necessary time or privacy in which to indulge. Nature's irony!

After age 18, a man's sexual functioning slowly declines. The most noticeable sign is that it becomes somewhat harder to get an erection, and the erections are less firm than they once were. Most men in their early 20s invariably wake up with erections. In their 40s and beyond, this occurs much less often. The time it takes to achieve orgasm also declines. Once an older man has ejaculated, it takes longer to achieve another erection. By age 50, most men are only having about half as much sex as they did in their younger years.

These changes do little to interfere with a man's ability to enjoy a varied and active sex life. It may take more effort, more foreplay, and more touching to achieve that erection, but so what? It's time well spent, if you ask me. Plus, there's a happy trade-off. Older men are generally "slower on the trigger." It takes them longer to get hard, but once they have an erection they're able to make love longer. Even when they don't get erections as often as they'd like, they learn more about using foreplay to stimulate themselves and their partners. Since women typically require more time to achieve orgasm than men, this "delay" often makes sex more satisfying for both of them.

Changes in Women

Now, the women's side. Women reach their sexual peaks—a time when they achieve orgasm most easily—much later than men, usually between the ages of 35 and 40. As estrogen levels decline in the years leading up to menopause, there's a corresponding decline in libido. Low levels of estrogen also result in a weakening of the vaginal muscles and a thinning of the vaginal walls. Loss of lubrication and difficulties with painful sex, or dyspareunia, become much more common.

Despite these changes, a woman's interest in sex, and her ability to enjoy it, persists. In surveys, more than 50% of women ages 60 and older say that a satisfying sexual relationship is important for their overall quality of life. The frequency of intercourse does diminish, but as I mentioned before, women in these older age groups approach their sexuality in more varied ways. A survey by the American Association of Retired Persons found that 73% of married older women engaged in kissing and sexual touching more than once a week. More than half had sexual intercourse with the same frequency, and 18% were having oral sex.

A woman's ability to have orgasms does decrease with age. Between the ages of 40 and 50, for example, 33% of women report that they always have an orgasm with their partner. Between the ages of 50 and 60, on the other hand, the percentage drops to 26. The interesting paradox is that despite the diminishing frequency of orgasms, older women are more satisfied with their sex lives than their younger counterparts. This is presumably because the emotional components of sex bring as much or more satisfaction than the fireworks. Indeed, 40% of women over age 50 feel that they're better lovers than they were when they were younger.

I still remember a patient I saw about 10 years ago. She was 78, recently widowed, and lusty as a goat. She was dating two men and, from what I could tell, was enjoying sex as much as, if not more than, she ever had. She admitted, however, that vaginal dryness was slowing her down. She enjoyed frequent intercourse, but it was painful. "Oral sex only goes so far," she complained.

Not so long ago, doctors probably would have dismissed her very reasonable complaint with an indifferent platitude, something along the lines of, "Slow down, you're not as young as you used to be." They gave the same kinds of useless (and cold-hearted) advice for all sorts of age-related problems, from knee pain to fatigue. I'm embarrassed to think that members of my profession not only allowed older adults to accept a diminished status in life, but actually encouraged it. Attitudes have changed, thank goodness, and there's a consensus among my colleagues in gerontology that there's no earthly reason for anyone to slow down when they don't have to. Quit having sex? What ridiculous advice!

Anyway, back to my patient. I sent her away with a prescription for estrogen cream, which restores vaginal strength. I also advised her to use a water-based lubricant prior to sex. When she came back to the office a month later, she told me that sex had become a lot more comfortable. "Three times a week!" she said, clapping her hands. I've continued to see her since then. She's now pushing 90, but she still has sex once or twice a week. She usually has orgasms, and she has no plans to marry again.

DEALING WITH CHANGES

Sexual intimacy is such an important part of long-term physical and emotional health that it's easy for doctors to oversimplify their advice to the point of absurdity. I'm guilty of it myself. On more than one occasion, I've found myself echoing the famous Nike slogan: "Just do it!" It's good advice, as far as it goes, but it's almost insulting to the millions of Americans who would love nothing better than to be sexually active, but who, for a variety of reasons, can't. Sad to say, sexual problems are common in men as well as women. They're a source of untold embarrassment and shame, and they contribute, directly or not, to a significant percentage of failed relationships.

The paradoxical thing is that the angst we feel about sexual problems is wildly disproportionate to the available solutions. For men and women both, most sexual difficulties—reduced libido, impotence, lack of lubrication, and so on—are readily treatable. To be sure, some sexual dysfunctions are deeply rooted in the psyche, and therapy—sometimes long-term and often expensive—may be the best way out. But these are the exceptions. Most problems can be resolved very quickly with a combination of over-the-counter products or prescription drugs, and perhaps a little common sense.

Healthy Body, Healthy Sex

Before I delve into the most common problems, it's worth stepping back for a moment to look at the normal sexual responses in men and women. All arousal starts in the brain. When the brain is stimulated, it sends chemical signals—in the forms of neuropeptide Y, vasointestinal polypeptide, and nitric oxide—through the central nervous system. The chemical rush is what creates the surge of arousal and allows the subsequent sexual activity. In men, these signals are simultaneously sent to the penis and prostate gland, promoting erection; in women, the signals that get the ball rolling go to the clitoris, vagina, and uterus, causing relaxation and lubrication.

Hormones play a key role in arousal. Estrogen, for example, promotes vaginal muscle tone and lubrication. Lubrication does more than make sex comfortable. It also makes the vagina somewhat acidic and less hospitable to yeast and other infections. When estrogen levels decline at menopause, the loss of lubrication can make sex less comfortable. Lower levels of estrogen also reduce libido and the ability to have orgasms.

We think of testosterone as a male hormone, but women have it too. Menopausal declines in testosterone can cause a decline in libido. For men, of course, testosterone is the key sexual hormone. But unlike women, men don't experience significant hormone declines. Testosterone levels do decrease with age, but this is unlikely to affect a man's ability to get aroused and have erections.

So that's pretty much how it works. You must have adequate levels of sex hormones to maintain an interest in, and the ability to have, sex. You need a healthy brain to trigger arousal and send the appropriate signals. And you need an intact nerve and blood supply and healthy tissues to respond to chemical signals. Problems in any one of these areas can result in reduced sex drive, impotence, loss of lubrication, and so on.

Don't Ignore Sexual Problems!

Despite our national fixation on sex, it's rarely the most important part of a successful marriage. At least, as long as the sex is working. But—and this is a big "but"—sexual problems can undermine even the most healthy and committed relationship. Sex is such a critical component of health that every physician should discuss it with patients. Unfortunately, doctors are no more comfortable discussing sex than anyone else. They'll certainly answer questions if you ask them directly, but they're less likely to bring up sexual issues during routine checkups.

I always ask my patients about sex, not only because changes in sexual activity may be a sign of other potentially serious problems, but because sex itself is such a powerful predictor of long-term health. If my patients aren't having sex, or if there have been changes in their usual sexual activities, I want to know about it. Most of my patients, not surprisingly, are reluctant to talk about sex, even if a particular problem is very much on their minds. What usually happens is that we'll spend half an hour or more discussing whatever health problem brought them in the door. Then, when they're about ready to leave, they'll spring something like, "Do you think Viagra will help me?" I often wonder if that was the real reason they came to the office. So we sit back down, and I try to find out what's going on behind those closed doors.

Please, do not ignore sexual issues! Don't give up and live with them. Talk to a doctor. It's crazy for any of us to be so embarrassed that we refuse to talk about this very important part of our lives. Remember what I said before: The vast majority of sex problems can be resolved, usually without an enormous investment in time or energy. It saddens me when I see people suffering unnecessarily. One of my patients, a man in his 70s, was frustrated because his wife didn't want to have sex. She isn't my patient, so I don't have a clue what her issues are. But I witnessed the ugly consequences when the man, after pursuing an affair (and getting caught), suddenly found himself in a marriage that had disintegrated beyond repair. When one partner in a marriage loses interest in sex, or for whatever reason is unable to have sex, the negative effects can be far-reaching. I certainly don't blame the woman in this case. It's possible that her reluctance to have sex was simply indicative of an unhappy marriage. But surely they could have done more.

Because sex is such a taboo issue in this country, people don't begin to realize how common sexual problems are. One study, for example, found that 87% of American women were concerned about their low interest in sex. About 83% had difficulty achieving orgasm, 74% had problems with lubrication, and 72% were concerned about pain. These numbers are astounding. Even though other studies have reported lower levels of sexual problems—a report in the *Journal of the American Medical Association*, for example, found that 43% of women ages 18 to 59 had some degree of sexual dysfunction—it's clear that a lot of us are having significant issues in the bedroom.

It's impossible in a short chapter to do justice to the enormous range of potential sexual problems and treatments, but here's a quick look at the main ones.

Sex and the Older Woman

Let's start with women's issues.

Reduced libido. It's by far the most common cause of sexual dysfunction in women. Almost anything can cause it: marital conflicts, depression, or physical problems, such as frequent urinary infections. Low levels of estrogen can certainly cause libido to plummet. A drop in testosterone, which promotes desire as well as lubrication and clitoral enlargement during arousal, is even more likely. Hormone levels are very easy to check, and they're just as easy to correct. If, on the other hand, the problem is related to boredom, things get a bit more challenging. Women who are no longer attracted to their partners, or are simply bored with their sexual routines, may need to add some spice: trying different sexual positions, watching erotic videos for ideas, and so on.

Arousal disorders. A woman may want to have sex, but find that she's not getting aroused the way she used to. This is very common in older women, and it's wonderfully easy to treat. Basically, women need to pay more attention to their own needs. The use of a lubricant will almost certainly help. Women should also insist on more foreplay and more direct clitoral stimulation, either with a finger (their own or their partner's) or a vibrator.

Difficulty achieving orgasm. Once again, the key is to maximize stimulation—and minimize inhibition! I've found that many women are much too passive in this regard. Don't wait for your partner to do the right thing. You have to take care of yourself. If this means indulging with a vibrator for half an hour before making love, go for it. You might benefit from Kegel exercises. You alternately squeeze and then relax the pelvic muscles, and repeat the exercise frequently throughout the day, or even during sex. Kegels can help promote orgasm in some women.

Vaginal pain or dryness. Whatever you do, don't quit having sex because of vaginal discomfort. It's among the easiest problems to treat. Many women do just fine by applying a comfortable, water-based lubricant before sex. Some may need a prescription estrogen cream. Others use both, usually with great success.

Sex and the Older Man

Now, for the male side of things. While men can and do suffer from loss of libido, the problem that gets the most attention, and provokes the most anxiety, is impotence, also known as erectile dysfunction. About 31% of men suffer from erection problems at some times in their lives, and it tends to get worse with advancing age. A man in his late 50s is three times more likely to have erection problems than a man in his 20s. After age 70, the incidence can reach 80%.

Until recently, doctors thought that most erection problems were "all in the head." Low levels of testosterone have also been blamed, although this rarely occurs in men under the age of 80. We generally evaluate testosterone levels in any man 70 years or older who has erection problems, but low testosterone rarely explains it. So what does cause it? The two most common culprits are inadequate blood supply or an interruption of the nerve signals that trigger erections. Let's look at blood flow first. The same fatty deposits that line the coronary arteries and increase the risk of heart disease also occur in the smaller blood vessels in the penis. Inadequate blood flow prevents the penis from getting hard. Nerve damage, by itself or in combination with blood flow problems, can also result in occasional or total impotence.

Earlier, I may have sounded a bit dismissive about the link between impotence and psychological issues. While so-called psychogenic impotence is no longer thought to be the main cause of erection difficulties, it can play a role. For example, some men have so many conflicts in their relationships that arousal is unlikely. Others worry so much about their ability to perform that they can't. This happens to nearly every man on occasion, especially those who have physical problems at the same time. As you can imagine, this can lead to a very uncomfortable cycle. A man who fails to get an erection will worry more the next time. The worry makes him less likely to succeed, which will lead to even more worry.

Men are extremely reluctant to talk to their doctors (or anyone else) about erection problems, but they should. In nearly all cases, a man can regain all or most of his ability to have an erection. The drug Viagra is one of the most exciting breakthroughs of recent years. It promotes blood flow into the penis during times of arousal, and studies show that it works in about 70% of cases. Best of all, it generally works as well in older men as in younger ones. It's also helpful for those with vascular problems, diabetes, and multiple sclerosis. It's even been shown to help men who have developed impotence following prostate surgery.

Most men who take Viagra won't experience serious side effects. Doctors discovered early on, however, that it may be harmful when it's combined with nitrates, drugs commonly used to treat heart disease. Some of my older patients, as a result, are reluctant to take Viagra because they've heard it's bad for the heart. Except for those taking medications, this doesn't seem to be the case. A recent study in the *Journal of the American Medical Association* found that Viagra appeared to be safe even in those with relatively severe coronary artery disease.

The older you are, and the worse the underlying physical problems—reduced blood flow or interrupted nerve signals—the less likely you are to be helped by Viagra. Ask your doctor if you'd benefit from injections of prostaglandin or papaverine into the penis. I know, it sounds painful and totally unsexy. But the needles are so small that most men hardly feel them, and the drugs produce strong, long-lasting erections.

Two other options are worth mentioning. There's a vacuum device that literally sucks blood into the penis. Once an erection occurs, a small rubber band is placed around the base of the penis to maintain the erection. The mechanical approach is off-putting to some men, but the machines do work quite well. If all else fails, your doctor may recommend surgery to implant an inflatable device inside the penis. When a man is ready for sex, all he has to do is press a pump implanted in the groin, and a wonderful erection springs to life. Men are advised to think long and hard before having the surgery, however. It destroys a man's natural ability to have an erection, so it's only recommended for those who can't be helped in any other way.

I've been focusing on the physical treatments for erection problems, but the emotional factors are big ones—if not in causing impotence, then in how you cope with it. Difficulty getting an erection, sad to say, is a natural part of maturity. It sometimes happens. Share your concerns with your partner. Don't hesitate to see it as an opportunity to strengthen your feelings of love and intimacy, and to engage in long and erotic foreplay. Your vulnerability may lead the way to even greater sexual tenderness and satisfaction.

MEDICINE'S SEXUAL SIDE EFFECTS

For men and women both, perhaps the most common correctable cause of sexual dysfunction is drugs. All of the issues we've talked about—problems with libido, erectile difficulties, and so on—can be caused by some of the most frequently used drugs in America. Because of the complex nature of sexual interest, arousal, and performance, it's not surprising that many, many drugs, with their multiple actions in the body, might cause trouble.

One of the first things I think about, when I see a patient who is having sexual problems, is whether one or more drugs might be responsible. I always ask patients to bring a complete list of all the prescription and over-the-counter medications they're taking, supplements and alternative medicines included. I enlist the help of the pharmacist I work with, and we look at each and every drug to see if it might be causing problems. If we identify one or more likely culprits, we brainstorm for better alternatives. The drug Wellbutrin, for example, is less likely to cause sexual problems than other antidepressants. ACE inhibitors are often a better choice than beta-blockers.

Here is a wonderful example of a true success story. One of my patients, a handsome, 67-year-old man, is married to one of the most exciting and voluptuous women I've ever met. He came to see me mainly because he was suffering from fatigue. In addition, he was profoundly depressed because he had lost the ability to get an erection. He had tried Viagra, but it didn't help.

There didn't seem to be anything wrong with him that would explain the sudden development of impotence. So I asked, as I always do, about the medications he was taking. It turned out he was taking gemfibrozil, one of the older cholesterol-lowering drugs—one that causes impotence in about 12% of men who take it. Even if he needed help lowering cholesterol (blood tests later revealed that he didn't), this wasn't the drug I would have chosen. In any event, I told him to quit taking it. Bingo. His fatigue lifted, and the next time I saw him, he gave me a wink and a smile.

And then there's my own story. I've mentioned that I had a heart attack some years back, and, coincidentally, I've also suffered from gen-

COMMON DRUGS WITH SEXUAL SIDE EFFECTS

Antidepressants
- Lithium
- SSRIs
  - Prozac
  - Paxil
  - Zoloft
  - Celexa
  - Effexor
- Tricyclic antidepressants
- Monoamine oxidase inhibitors

Antihypertensives
- Beta blockers
  Atenolol and metoprolol
- Cardura
- Clonidine
- Hytrin
- Methyldopa
- Reserpine

Antipsychotics
- Haldol
- Risperdal
- Zyprexa

Diuretics
- Spironolactone

Cardiac Drugs and Cholesterol-Lowering Agents
- Digoxin
- Gemfibrozil (Lopid)
- Clofibrate

Gastrointestinal drugs
- Reglan
- Tagamet

Hormones
- Estrogen and progesterone
- Proscar
- Corticosteroids
- Lupron (antitestosterone)
- Danazol (Danocrine)

Nonsteroidal anti-inflammatory drugs (NSAIDs)

Sedatives and tranquilizers
- Phenothiazines
- Valium and Librium
- Barbiturates

eralized muscle pain, especially in my chest. After the heart attack, I had a hard time distinguishing muscle pain from heart pain, which led to more than a few panicky moments. My doctor thought the muscle pain might be caused by fibromyalgia. To relieve it, she gave me amitriptyline, an antidepressant that made my tongue so dry I literally had to peel it off the roof of my mouth in the morning. When I insisted on another drug, she recommended the antidepressant Paxil. It reduced the muscle pain, all right, but it also made my penis about as responsive as a lump of lead. I stopped taking it, and within three weeks I was back to normal. I decided to just live with the muscle pain—much better than that particular side effect.

The more I've learned about the wonderfully vibrant sex lives of many of my patients, the more I'm saddened by the negative, stereotypical views that permeate our culture. Just today, my daughter said, "Grandma having sex—that's disgusting." Well, she's 17. She can't imagine that anyone old enough to be a grandparent—or a parent, for that matter—could possibly have sexual desires and longings, much less act upon them. But every time I see my mother, she's almost glowing with happiness. I bet her great sex life has something to do with it.

Not all of us are this lucky, of course. If your sex life isn't as good as you'd like it to be, I strongly encourage you to discuss the issues, openly and honestly, with your doctor. If you don't get clear, helpful answers, find another doctor. Remember what I said earlier: Most sex problems can be corrected without a great deal of effort. At the same time, don't let embarrassment hold you back. Experiment. Try new positions. Fill your mind—or your partner's—with pleasant fantasies. Do whatever it takes to cultivate this wonderful side of yourself.

One of the reasons that I so adore my mother's lusty approach to life is that it suggests that we, the baby boomers, have a rosier sexual future than we might think. Those of us who are sexually active now are more likely to be sexually active later. What we lose in frequency we'll more than make up for in variety and intimacy. We'll make love longer, and we'll make love better. And I truly like the idea that one of the rewards of getting older is to shed more inhibitions and to be truly wild in bed.

So here's to the future—I can hardly wait.

CHAPTER NINE

*"I've been out with a lot of really nice gentlemen since I
moved here. Being older has its benefits when it comes to sex,
you know. Since I don't have to worry about birth control
anymore, there's no messing with diaphragms, or condoms, or
gels, or anything..."*   *—Sylvia, age 61*

STDs Don't
Discriminate

I don't think I'm naïve about the sexual behavior of my patients.
Anyone who works in geriatric medicine learns pretty quickly that
the desire for sex, along with the urge to experiment and try new
things, doesn't suddenly evaporate at retirement age. The older people
who are my patients may not get around as well as they used to, but their
libidos, judging from what they tell me, are alive and well.

For a while I admired all of this playful exuberance, but the medical
realities are too serious to be ignored. "Safe sex" is a mantra among
younger adults, but the message doesn't seem to be getting through to
the senior set. For some reason, common sense—and condoms—goes
out the window when men and women date people of their own age.
National surveys involving thousands of older adults consistently show
that about 93% of older adults *never* use condoms. They seem to think

that sexually transmitted diseases are a nonissue for them and their peers.

The opposite, I'm sad to say, is true. Doctors don't talk a lot about it, but there's been a startling rise in sexually transmitted diseases (STDs) in those 50 years and older. Researchers recently found that 10% of people in these upper age groups had one or more risk factors—for example, multiple sex partners or having unprotected sex with someone who has multiple sex partners—for getting an STD.

The STDs clearly on the rise in older adults are HIV (the deadly virus that causes AIDS), human papilloma virus (HPV), and hepatitis C. HPV is bothersome and it does increase the risk of cervical cancer, but you can live with it. HIV and hepatitis C, on the other hand, are potentially deadly. New infections of syphilis and gonorrhea are also on the rise in older adults.

Everyone, doctors as well as patients, has to start taking these diseases more seriously. They can be prevented, but only if people get it into their heads that age and maturity provide no protection. If anything, older people may be *more* at risk for getting STDs. And when they get them, they suffer the effects much more drastically than someone younger.

What people need to understand is that older, sexually active people are more susceptible to STDs, and HIV in particular. The vaginal tissues in older women lose elasticity and are more vulnerable to tears, thereby increasing the risk that malignant viruses can get into the bloodstream. In addition, older people have weaker immunity to begin with, which means that their immune system is less able to mount a robust response to early infection with any given STD. In the case of HIV infection, once AIDS-related illnesses develop, older people tend to get sicker and recover more slowly. A number of studies have shown that HIV in older adults has a shorter incubation time before it progresses to full-blown

AIDS. In those under age 50, only 12% die within a month of the diagnosis. *In those 80 and over, 40% die within a month of diagnosis.*

A SHAMEFUL SILENCE

The relatively tame stories I hear in my office didn't prepare me for the out-and-out debauchery that I've witnessed on visits to retirement communities in Arizona and elsewhere. "My God," I said to my wife one day. "These people are as randy as goats!"

I kept coming across newspaper stories about lusty couples—in their 70s and 80s, mind you—who had been arrested for lewd behavior on park benches, in parked cars, and just about everywhere else. In areas with large populations of older adults, it's not uncommon to see bumper stickers that sport the admonishing message, "Get a room!" I also heard a lot of references to "condo cowboys." As you'd expect, healthy men who are active in the dating scene are at a premium in these upper age groups. In some retirement communities, women outnumber men by about five to one, and believe me, the guys were making the most of it. If the barroom conversations I overheard had a kernel of truth to them—and I suspect they did—men in their 70s and 80s were routinely having sex with two or more women a week.

You would think that doctors would be all over the issue of rising STDs in the older set. Yet fewer than 10% of physicians discuss STDs with older patients. This is partly due to embarrassment. Doctors are no more comfortable talking about sex than anyone else, and they're loath to intrude into peoples' private lives. Yet they somehow manage to broach the subject with younger patients. Why not with older folks? I suspect it's because doctors (like the rest of our society) have a hard time thinking of older adults as sexual beings. The assumption is that seniors don't have sex, or at least don't engage in adventuresome (or risky) sex. Frankly, we have our heads in the sand. An epidemic is raging, and no one's talking about it.

I see a lot of STDs in my practice, and the issue does make me little uncomfortable. A few days ago I evaluated a 69-year-old woman with genital herpes. The diagnosis had originally been made by a gynecologist, who gave her a prescription for Famvir, an antiviral drug that suppresses, but doesn't eliminate, the virus. What the doctor neglected to do was explain to the woman that this form of herpes is always transmitted sexually. I can understand the doctor's urge to sidestep the issue. I wasn't eager myself to delve into the woman's private life and suggest that she (or her husband) had some sexual issues to discuss. But people need to know when their behavior is getting them into trouble. We're not shy about pointing the finger at other health-threatening lifestyle issues, like the overconsumption of fatty foods or a lack of exercise. We have to do the same thing for STDs, regardless of how much emotional turmoil the diagnosis invariably entails.

When I told the woman that herpes is caused by sexual contact, she got a puzzled look on her face. "Impossible," she said—she had always been faithful to her husband of 47 years. After a brief pause, she asked the obvious question. Did this mean her husband had been unfaithful? What a terrible question to have to answer! I found myself envying her gynecologist, who took the easy—if medically irresponsible—way out. I answered her question indirectly by explaining how genital herpes is spread. When I told her that the symptoms can appear intermittently for years or decades after the initial exposure, her mood brightened somewhat. She had experienced minor symptoms over the years, nothing serious enough to tell her doctor about, but bothersome all the same. It was possible, she suggested, that she'd been infected with the virus many years before.

The thought gave her comfort, for obvious reasons, but given the length of time they'd been married, it was likely that one or both of them had strayed at some point. I didn't push the issue. The last thing I wanted to do was make her feel worse than she already did. But I did make sure she fully understood the issues involved, if only so she could take the necessary precautions to prevent someone else from getting infected.

HIV AND AIDS

AIDS is arguably the most devastating disease in human history. Caused by HIV, AIDS essentially destroys the immune system and leaves people vulnerable to cancer and a host of infectious diseases. In the United States, AIDS has disproportionately affected young gay men and intravenous drug users, but no one should be lulled into thinking they're immune. Worldwide, AIDS affects many more heterosexuals than homosexuals, and the incidence among older adults is skyrocketing. Between 10 and 16% of all new cases of HIV are diagnosed in people age 50 and older. HIV infection in this group jumped 138% between 1993 and 2000. In just the last five years, the incidence of HIV in women age 50 and older has increased 40%. In the United States, the incidence of HIV is increasing most rapidly in heterosexual men and women over the age of 50.

Not Just a Disease of the Young

Despite the trends, people continue to think of AIDS as a young person's disease. This misconception has had disastrous consequences. People who are convinced that AIDS can't happen to them don't think to get tested. Since the virus can linger in the body for as long as a decade without causing symptoms, there's ample time and opportunity for them to unknowingly pass it onto to others.

Doctors are just as likely as patients to overlook AIDS in older adults. Scientists recently reported that 5% of 60-year-old patients who died at Harlem Hospital in New York City were HIV-positive. Yet in none of these cases was HIV diagnosed; doctors simply didn't think to test for it. Similarly, older patients who are diagnosed with syphilis are rarely screened for HIV. This is a dangerous omission because syphilis greatly increases the risk of HIV transmission.

It's a Catch-22 situation. Older patients with HIV do dramatically better when they're diagnosed at the earliest possible time. And yet, doctors often neglect to test for the disease because they aren't looking for it. To be fair, many of the early symptoms of HIV infection—fatigue, weight loss, and anemia, for example—are somewhat vague and nonspecific. But even when patients come in with symptoms that are the hallmarks of AIDS, such as thrush (a fungal infection), tuberculosis, or the reactivation of old shingles infections, their doctor may not think to look for AIDS. So much time can pass before the disease is finally diagnosed that the available treatments are much less effective.

As with all sexually transmitted diseases, there's a great deal of denial surrounding AIDS. The disease is spread primarily by sexual contact, less often by the intermingling of contaminated blood. Yet about 26% of people 50 years and older who are newly diagnosed with HIV claim that they have no risk factors for getting the disease. I suppose some people really don't know what causes AIDS. Most of the time, I'm sure, people simply don't want to admit to the things they've done to put themselves at risk.

Just to put the record straight: HIV is usually transmitted sexually. Sexual intercourse is the main mode of transmission, although oral sex isn't without risk. People who are newly infected with HIV will usually have enlarged lymph nodes and flu-like symptoms. The immune system initially kills virus particles in the blood, but some virus particles sur-vive and replicate inside specialized immune cells. About 10 to 12 years after the initial infection, the virus "load" is high enough that it starts causing symptoms, such as pneumonia, fungal infections, cancers, and even dementia.

Everyone who is at risk—those who have had multiple sex partners or have had sex without condoms, or have used (or been with someone who used) intravenous drugs—should get tested for HIV. Early detec-tion is critical because there are a number of antiviral drugs that can suppress the virus for many, many years. There isn't a cure for AIDS, but it's often possible to reduce viral loads to virtually undetectable levels.

Treatment for AIDS

The standard treatment for HIV is to give drug "cocktails" known as HAART, or highly active antiretroviral therapy. The drugs aren't perfect, but they've dramatically increased survival rates for those with HIV or AIDS—so much so, in fact, that AIDS is no longer among the top ten causes of death in the United States. Giving drugs in combination means that the virus can be attacked at different stages of its replication cycle. There are many drugs available for fighting HIV, but they all fall into two main categories: nucleoside reverse transcriptase inhibitors, which pre-vent the virus from hijacking the DNA of normal cells; and protease inhibitors, which block an enzyme that the virus needs to replicate.

I want to emphasize that HAART does not cure AIDS. It does not prevent transmission of the disease. And it's hardly a picnic. The drugs are expensive, and they have to be taken according to very strict sched-ules. Missing even a few doses can allow the virus to rebound in record time. Also, nearly everyone who takes the drugs has side effects. Nau-sea and diarrhea are common. The therapy also may cause an unusual distribution of body fat; the face and arms may become unusually thin, while the neck and abdomen enlarge dramatically.

The drugs for HIV and AIDS are an impressive scientific breakthrough. They've transformed AIDS from an automatic death sentence into a chronic, slowly progressing disease that can be managed for many years. But the very success of these drugs has lulled people into complacency. Fewer and fewer people of all age groups are practicing safe sex, which has allowed HIV to spread much farther and faster than it should. If you're 50 or older and are sexually active, you're very much at risk. Please, take it seriously.

HUMAN PAPILLOMA VIRUS

Human papilloma virus is far and away the most common STD in the United States. There are a hundred different HPV viruses, thirty of which are spread sexually. It's estimated that more than 40 million Americans are infected with HPV. The virus is so ubiquitous, and so easily spread, that nearly everyone who's sexually active has probably been exposed to it at some point. It tends to crop up first in young people, simply because they're the ones who are most likely to be dating or having sex with new partners. But HPV can also make its unwelcome appearance in older adults. This often happens after divorce or the death of a spouse, when men and women are thrust back into the dating scene after being away from it for many years.

Disconcerting Warts

I certainly see a great deal of HPV in my practice. What brings people with this disease into my office is the disconcerting discovery of a wart or warts that crop up near or on the genitals. In women, the warts can spread into the vaginal opening or onto the cervix. Men tend to get the warts on the tip or shaft of the penis. The warts are highly infectious. If you have sex with someone who has genital warts, you have about a 60% chance of getting them yourself within three months. Keep in mind that the warts aren't always limited to the genital area. People who have oral sex with an infected partner will sometimes get warts on the esophagus.

One of the hardest jobs of any physician, I think, is telling patients, especially older, more conservative patients, that their condition, whatever it is, was caused by sexual contact. Some years ago, a good friend of mine confided that she had a terrible case of genital warts. The warts were extensive, and she had been seeing her gynecologist every week to have them removed. She seemed to have no idea that genital warts are a sexually transmitted disease. Since she'd been married for decades, and the warts had only recently appeared, it was obvious that either she or her husband had strayed outside the marriage. Although I silently cursed her physician for not explaining things clearly, I was grateful that I didn't have to be the one to break the news.

Whether or not warts are present, HPV isn't painful. Unless you actually see the warts, which can spontaneously appear and disappear throughout your life, you won't even know you're infected. This is why the disease is so widespread, and it's also why it can cause serious complications.

HPV and Cervical Cancer

Men with HPV don't have much to worry about. But in women, infection with the virus has been linked to cancer of the cervix, a disease that carries a much worse prognosis when it's diagnosed in women 65 years or older. The survival rate of cervical cancer in women under age 45 is 70%; in those 65 or older, the survival rate drops to 30%.

The warts caused by HPV are easy to spot during routine exams. Doctors apply a vinegar solution to suspicious areas. The warts whiten more than the surrounding areas, making them easy to recognize. Once you know you have warts, the treatment is straightforward. A number of chemical liquids, including podophyllin and trichloroacetic acid, will destroy warts on contact. The FDA recently approved a cream called Aldara, which is also effective. The warts can also be removed by applying liquid nitrogen, in a procedure called cryotherapy. The nitrogen freezes the warts and causes them to die and slough off.

Because women infected with HPV have a high risk of cervical cancer, they must have regular Pap smears. One reassuring point is that not all strains of HPV cause cervical cancer, and only about 10% of women exposed to the virus will go on to develop cervical cancer. In fact, the strains of HPV that cause cancer are the ones less likely to form warts. So don't panic if you (or your doctor) discovers genital warts. You will need a Pap smear, but that's a test you should be getting in any event.

HEPATITIS C

For a long time, hepatitis C was virtually ignored by the public health community. A viral infection, it can linger in the body, undiagnosed, for decades before causing symptoms. Most people who get hepatitis C aren't aware of how they got it, how long they've had it, or what, if anything, can be done to treat it.

And yet, the hepatitis C virus (HCV) affects some 200 million people worldwide, far more than are infected with the AIDS virus. In the United States alone, doctors have identified more than 5 million cases of HCV, and many more cases undoubtedly exist beneath the radar. It can be a terrible infection. While 15 to 20% of those infected with HCV never develop serious symptoms, 80 to 85% go on to develop chronic hepatitis, or liver inflammation. Twenty percent of those who have chronic hepatitis will go on to develop cirrhosis, or liver damage, within 20 years. Of these, fully half will suffer irreparable liver damage or liver cancer.

For a long time, the main cause of HCV was blood transfusions. Tests to detect tainted blood have been widespread since 1985, so this mode of transmission has been all but eliminated. Yet millions of people are still being infected, often because of intravenous drug use, but also because of sexual activity with an infected partner. Doctors estimate that anywhere from 1 to 10% of HCV infections occur in people with multiple sex partners. Another risk factor is infection with genital herpes or other STDs: They seem to aid in the transmission of HCV.

Now that we can screen blood for HCV, blood transfusions are unlikely to spread the disease. What this means, of course, is that people who are infected probably got it by sexual contact or intravenous drug use. Older adults, I'm afraid, are extremely vulnerable. The vaginal tissue gets weaker and thinner with age, and the almost inevitable tears provide an easy gateway for the virus. Studies suggest that sexual contact accounts for about 16% of HCV infections. Older people also have less robust immune systems and liver function, which can make the course of the disease more serious.

I see quite a bit of HCV in my practice. It's usually spotted (or at least suspected) during routine liver function tests. When the tests are abnormal, we always test for the HCV virus. All too often, I'm afraid, we find it. Just recently, I saw a man in his 60s with quite severe liver disease caused by HCV. Apparently his wife was exposed to the virus in the 1960s (before blood screening tests were available) while getting a blood transfusion during heart surgery, and she passed it on to him.

For now, there isn't a reliable cure for HCV. Two drugs, interferon-A and ribavirin, can sometimes normalize liver function and eradicate HCV particles from the blood. In most cases, however, the virus manages to survive and the infection comes right back. For those with severe liver damage, a transplant is the only real option.

PREVENTING STDS

So here we are, men and women ages 50 and older, still very interested in and enjoying sex. Many of us came of age long before sexual openness—and sexual risks—were a part of daily life. In retrospect, the sexual revolution of the 1960s seems pretty tame, if for no other reason than that the worst it had to offer was the occasional encounter with gonorrhea or syphilis. Not a pleasant experience, to be sure, but one that was easily managed. Today, we face the frightening reality of AIDS and hepatitis C, potentially deadly diseases without cures.

I recently heard about a 55-year-old woman who was diagnosed with HIV after six months in a monogamous second marriage. She and her husband had quit using condoms, as most couples do. It wasn't until her husband developed AIDS that she realized that she, too, was probably infected. It's a tragic story, but one that illustrates just how careful we all have to be.

In the pages above, I focused on AIDS, hepatitis C, and human papilloma virus because they pose the greatest threat and are at such epidemic proportions that they can truly be called a crisis. But other STDs, among them herpes simplex, chlamydia, gonorrhea, and syphilis, are also frighteningly common in older adults. What all STDs have in common is that they're spread by sexual contact, and, more important, can all be prevented. This last point tends to get overlooked among older adults, who believe, wrongly, that they're somehow more immune than younger folks. Until safe sex is practiced uniformly across all age groups, the incidence of these diseases is going to keep rising.

Who's most at risk for getting infected? People who:

• Are sexually active and don't use latex condoms.

• Are unaware of their partners' sex or drug histories.

• Are injecting drugs, sharing needles, or otherwise coming into contact with infected blood.

• Had a blood transfusion between 1978 and 1985, or who had a blood transfusion in another country.

It's all pretty straightforward, and yet I've found, again and again, that many of my patients are totally unfamiliar with how these diseases are spread, and misconceptions abound. There are still people who won't enter a room if someone infected with HIV is present. They won't shake hands, and they certainly won't hug or kiss. All I can do is sigh. STDs are only caused by sexual contact or the intermingling of blood. Not by kissing. Not by hugging. Not by sitting on a motel toilet seat. These diseases are scary enough by themselves. We don't have to make them scarier with bad information.

Of course, just as people imagine risks where there aren't any, they also ignore risks that are very much present. Both HIV and hepatitis C, for example, are frequently caused by contact with infected blood. Forget blood from transfusions—that's been taken care of. Other blood sources are now the problem. Research has suggested, for example, that tattoo artists who don't adequately sterilize their equipment may be transmitting hepatitis C. More commonly, the sharing of toothbrushes and razors is a real concern—a bit of fatherly advice that really shocked my 21-year-old daughter. "We all share razors at college," she said.

I know they do. I also know that tiny razor nicks, too small to see or feel, are more than enough to transmit hepatitis C. So does sharing a toothbrush. You might not see your gums bleeding, but they do it all the time. That blood is just as dangerous as having sex without a condom. Yet my daughter and her friends, who are better versed in STDs and preventive strategies than most older adults, don't have a clue that they might be exposing themselves to devastating illnesses.

I hate to say it, but for those of us in our 50s or older, it's probably too late to do anything about HPV. If you were sexually active 20, 30, or 40 years ago, you were almost certainly infected. This doesn't mean, however, that you should feel free to infect others. No one loves using condoms, but for now, they provide the best protection for those who are sexually active.

I do my best not to moralize to my patients. I'm well aware that my approach to sex and relationships is unlikely to be the same as theirs. But sometimes a little moralizing is part and parcel of good public health. Want to avoid STDs? A good place to start is getting to know and trust the people you hope to be sexually involved with. Learn about their history—sexual and otherwise. Always be wary of casual sex and one-night stands. You might have a wonderful time, but if you don't know, *really know*, who the person is, the risks are just too high.

Let's assume that you're in a new relationship, or have just started dating someone and you think a relationship is possible. Let me give some advice:

Don't be embarrassed to discuss STDs. Ask about your partner's sexual history. Were there a lot of different partners? Was he or she ever treated for genital warts or herpes? A history of STDs doesn't preclude a solid relationship by any means, but you do need to know what your risks are, and whether you'll need to take precautions.

Ask your partner to join you in getting tested for HIV and hepatitis C. It's not romantic, but it can keep you safe.

Always, and I mean *always,* **have sex with a latex condom** in the early stages of a relationship. Using a spermicide in combination with a condom gives even more protection.

How long do you have to use condoms? The usual advice is to use them until you've been in a monogamous relationship for six months. After six months, get tested for HIV and hepatitis C. If you're both clear, use condoms for another six months, then get tested again. At that point you can give up the condoms, as long as the relationship stays monogamous.

Never, ever have unprotected sex if your partner has genital warts. You *will* be infected.

Never have unprotected sex with someone who has active herpes.

For women: Schedule an annual Pap smear, especially if you've had sex with a new partner. Don't wait for warts to appear: Most women who develop HPV-related malignancies never get the warts.

Don't share toothbrushes or razors. (My daughter has promised that she will never share a razor with anyone again.)

Studies have clearly shown that couples in committed, monogamous relationships have more frequent, more satisfying sex than those who are single. Monogamous relationships aren't for everyone, I know, but do keep the risks of having multiple partners in mind in order to better protect yourself. The more sexual partners you have, the greater your risk of getting infected. It's always better, and safer, to get to know potential lovers and take the time to develop intimacy, love, and commitment.

CHAPTER TEN

"I read about these growth hormone injections. Had trouble getting them in the United States, but fortunately I have a friend who buys the vials for me in Tijuana. I feel great, but I'm worried about these really bad headaches and this pain in my hand."

—Ted, age 56

ANTI-AGING HYPE: ONLY A KERNEL OF TRUTH

I can't count the number of patients who have said to me, more or less in jest, "What can I take for old age?" or "Do whatever you can to make me young again." Their comments reveal the universal and, to me, very touching desire for youth. None of us wants to get old. We want to live forever, to stay fit, attractive, and mentally agile throughout our lives. And that's not just a generality: Congressional committees estimate that Americans spend as much as *$30 billion* annually on products and medical services that purportedly delay the aging process.

ON THE TRAIL TO THE FOUNTAIN OF YOUTH

In just the last decade or so, we've learned a great deal about the biology of aging. For the first time in scientific history, we're getting a handle on how cells age, how the machinery inside cells undergoes changes that lead to age-related diseases and eventually death. A number of reputable researchers have proposed specific strategies that could *theoretically* slow the aging process. These strategies aren't proven, and their practical applications are a long way off. But I have to say, we've already uncovered enough evidence to suggest that we might just find the Fountain (or Fountains) of Youth after all.

I'm not talking about eternal life, understand. I think it's reasonable to speculate that, in the fullness of time, advances in technology may give us the tools to extend human life well beyond our current boundaries—perhaps to 160 years or more. Even if we don't discover ways to actually slow (or stop) the aging process, it's entirely reasonable to speculate that we may find ways, at the cellular level, to stop many of the diseases associated with aging. In other words, anti-aging therapies of the future may or may not prolong life, but they'll almost certainly allow us to stay healthier throughout our life spans. And who knows? Maybe it really will be possible to slow the rate at which we age and, eventually, die.

"LONGEVITY MEDICINE": DUBIOUS AND COSTLY

Lifespans of 160 years or more are far, far in the future. But you wouldn't know it from the frantic sales pitches from supplement manufacturers and, I'm sad to say, too many of my medical colleagues. The medical fringes are increasingly occupied by an anti-aging contingent, physicians who claim that they have the ability, now, to retard the aging process. The American Academy of Anti-Aging Medicine, with a membership of 10,000 physicians, is one of the driving forces of so-called longevity medicine. Don't be fooled by the impressive-sounding title. "Longevity medicine" is not a recognized discipline within the mainstream medical community. Unlike other medical specialties—orthopedics, say, or internal medicine—doctors in this field aren't required to take courses specific to their subject. Any doctor who wants to launch an "anti-aging" practice under the auspices of this group only has to read a study guide and pass oral and written examinations.

I don't doubt that many of the physicians who bill themselves as anti-aging specialists are sincere, knowledgeable, caring professionals. But I also think they're jumping the gun way too soon, and there's more than a slight whiff of opportunism in the whole business that makes me uneasy. If you think visits to regular doctors are expensive, check out the price tag for seeing an doctor in an anti-aging clinic. A single visit, admittedly one that includes an exhaustive physical examination, can cost as much as $2000. I suppose that's a pittance if you're convinced that the reward will be the preservation—or even the recapture—of elusive youthful energy and sexual vigor.

There is, thankfully, a great deal of professional concern about what these anti-aging physicians are doing. The American Association of Retired Persons (AARP) has raised strong warnings about the practice of anti-aging medicine. Senator John Breaux of Louisiana, chair of the Senate Select Committee on Aging, has referred to "Twenty-first century snake oil salesmen." Dr. Jay Olshansky of the University of Illinois, Chicago, circulated a position paper, signed by 51 of the country's most eminent scientists, that warned about the hype of anti-aging remedies. "Anyone who claims they can stop or reverse the aging process is lying to you, even if they are a doctor," Dr. Olshansky wrote. "Anti-aging medicine is an industry intended to make money for those who are selling these products." Harsh words, to be sure. I believe Dr. Olshansky is right when he says there's no current evidence to support their medical practices.

THE TRUE SCIENCE BEHIND THE SNAKE OIL

In the following pages, I'm going to take a look at the main theories that attempt to explain the biology of aging. This isn't hucksterism by any means. It's legitimate science with a great deal of research behind it. Just remember the key caveat: *Theories aren't facts.* Something can be plausible without being true. To put it bluntly, there's no such thing as anti-aging medicine at this time. Anyone who says otherwise isn't telling the whole truth. Keep that in mind as you read on.

Calorie Restriction

Scientists have known for a long time that animals given low-calorie diets live longer. When animals are given about a third less calories than normal, their maximum life expectancy jumps by about 30%. That's not small potatoes. If the same thing were true in humans, cutting about 600 calories a day out of the average female diet would extend life expectancy from the current 83 years to an average of 100 years. The maximum life spans of humans could potentially increase from 120 years to 144 years!

Forget the issue of longevity for a moment. Apart from the fact that laboratory animals given these diets live longer, they also stay healthier.

Mice, for example, frequently die of kidney disease. But when their food intake is restricted, the incidence of kidney disease drops significantly. They're also less likely to get cancer, and if they do, it comes at a later age. Just about every marker of aging in these animals seems to be delayed. Calorie-restricted mice stay healthy for a very long time. Then, when they're much older than average, they gradually lose weight, get less active, and eventually lie down in a corner and die peacefully. Autopsies generally don't reveal a specific cause of death. There's no evidence of heart, lung or kidney failure, and no cancers can be identified. Sounds pretty good.

An Elusive Connection

The connection between low-calorie diets and advanced age is still elusive. We do know that cells throughout the body gradually lose their ability to neutralize toxic chemicals, and age-related changes in metabolism cause cells to function less efficiently. It's thought that restricting calories somehow makes cells more robust and more resistant to environmental assaults.

Recent research on monkeys has found similar results. So it's possible, but by no means certain, that humans could experience the same benefits. Then again, we might not. Scientists often fall into the trap of extrapolating the results of animal studies to humans. Sometimes it works out, sometimes it doesn't. Let's face it, we aren't mice. If we were, I could say with some certainty that one of the secrets of living longer, possibly much longer, would be to eat a lot less.

But would you really want to try this? Few of us, I think, would voluntarily forego a third of our daily calories for the rest of our lives. We simply don't have the stamina, or the desire, to go hungry all the time. I hate to say it, but the mice on these calorie-restricted diets aren't happy mice. They're overly active and agitated, and they're always hungry, which makes them pretty grumpy. Researchers on the study say the mice are always trying to bite the hands that *aren't* feeding them. Not much of a quality of life, I'm afraid. So even though it's theoretically possible that severe calorie restriction prolongs lifespan, it's not something that's practical in real life.

Antioxidants

You're probably familiar with the antioxidant theory of aging. It's been kicking around for about 50 years, but it's only in the last decade that it's really picked up steam. Millions of Americans routinely take vitamin E or other antioxidant supplements before they've had their morning coffee, and an increasing number of physicians routinely advise patients to take them—not to treat specific problems, but as an overall strategy for preventing disease and possibly extending life.

Marauding Free Radicals and Cellular Damage

There's a great deal of evidence that lifelong cellular damage is at the heart of age-related diseases. It may be at the heart of aging itself. What causes cellular damage? Often it's environmental. Exposure to air pollution, chemicals in water, background radiation, or even excessive sunshine can permanently damage the body's cells. But environmental factors play a relatively small role in cellular aging. The main assault comes from the body itself.

As cells go about their normal metabolic processes, they produce superoxide, hydroxyl radicals, and hydrogen peroxide, toxic byproducts known collectively as free radicals. Free radicals are highly unstable molecules that are missing an electron. They careen through the body like pinballs, grabbing electrons from other cells. In the process of ripping away electrons, they damage the cells—and create more free radicals in the process. Unless this free radical cascade is stopped, millions of cells in the brain, blood vessels, and other parts of the body will suffer irreparable damage.

The body has natural defenses against free radicals. It produces an enzyme called superoxide dismutase, which sacrifices its own electrons to the marauding free radicals. Once free radicals satisfy their need for electrons, the body's cells no longer come under assault. Here's the rub. The concentration of superoxide dismutase and other protective enzymes decline with age. This allows the concentration of free radicals, and the corresponding cellular damage, to increase. Multiply this by years and decades, and there may be profound damage to cell membranes, cellular proteins, and metabolic cellular components called mitochondria. Free radicals also damage the DNA inside cells, which reduces the cells' ability to divide and also increases the risk of cell mutations that give rise to cancers. Free radicals have been linked to just about every major disease, from heart disease and cancer to cataracts and Alzheimer's disease.

The True Value of Vitamins

Let's get back to vitamin E. Like superoxide dismutase and other antioxidant nutrients, such as vitamin C, selenium, and beta-carotene, it sacrifices its own electrons and provides a kind of protective barrier between free radicals and the vulnerable cells. The evidence is overwhelming that getting enough antioxidants in the diet (or possibly from supplements) can help prevent many chronic diseases. Research has shown, for example, that people who have had one heart attack can reduce their risk of a second heart attack by 30% when they take 800 IU of vitamin E daily. Preliminary studies suggest that people who take vitamin E regularly are up to 50% less likely to get Alzheimer's disease.

Okay, that's the theoretical background. Now, what about the claims in the anti-aging community that the use of vitamins or other antioxidants can extend life? I have to say, it makes intuitive sense. Laboratory studies show that animals that have been bred to have a high concentration of genes that produce the antioxidant superoxide dismutase live longer than those with lower concentrations. Similarly, scientists can shorten the lifespan of animals by breeding them for low superoxide dismutase production.

But so far, there's absolutely no evidence that people who take vitamin E or other antioxidant supplements live longer than those who don't. Nor have animal studies shown that antioxidants prolong life. That's the bottom line. These nutrients may be important for health. They may delay or prevent chronic diseases. But they haven't been shown to stop any of the cellular changes that are thought to be linked to aging itself.

Still, I'm excited by the possibility that antioxidant research may lead to the discovery of new compounds that will fulfill the promises of anti-aging proponents. Maybe we will eventually create a drug that enhances the natural protective powers of superoxide dismutase, or in some other fashion reduces cellular damage that's potentially at the heart of memory loss, low energy, heart disease, or other conditions associated with aging. But we haven't achieved this yet. Nor, for that matter, are we even sure that free radical damage plays a significant role in the aging process. It's a good theory, but it's not a fact.

If you aren't getting enough vitamins and minerals in your diet—and the majority of Americans aren't—go ahead and take a nutritional supplement. If you have risk factors for heart disease, or if you already have it, I do advise taking vitamin E. Vitamin C might be helpful if you have a cold, and it's certainly reasonable to take supplemental doses if you're a smoker because smoking robs the body of vitamin C. But should you bother taking these or other nutrients as part of an "anti-aging" regimen? Nah. Why should you? We aren't even sure what's behind the aging process. Cellular oxidation might—or might not—be one factor. Frankly, I think it's irresponsible of physicians to recommend taking high doses of supplements, which haven't been proven to work—and may even be dangerous, to boot, in excessive doses—to curtail a biological process that hasn't been proven to be hazardous.

Improved Immunity

One of the most exciting theories to emerge from research on the biology of aging is that gradual declines in immunity may be responsible for the majority of age-related diseases. It makes sense. The immune system is designed to recognize and destroy anything that's foreign—viruses, bacteria, even cancer cells. Young people have very strong immune systems. Should abnormal, cancerous cells develop, their immune systems are more likely than not to recognize and destroy them. This doesn't happen as readily in the elderly. Immunity declines over time, which is why older adults get more serious infections and are more likely to get cancer.

Thymosin and Other "Glandulars"

Age-related declines in immunity are largely due to changes in the thymus gland. Located closed to the heart, the thymus produces a number of hormones, among them thymosin, a hormone that regulates the maturation of infection-fighting immune cells called T cells. By the time you reach age 50, the thymus gland is about 15% of the size it was at birth, and there's a corresponding decline in levels of thymosin. This in turn makes us more vulnerable to bacterial and viral infections as well as to cancer.

Age is also accompanied by a decrease in immune cells called B cells. These cells recognize proteins on the membranes of bacteria, viruses, and cancer cells, and produce antibodies in response. Antibodies attach to these foreign cells and target them for destruction by still other immune cells. When B cells decline, the body loses its ability to recognize potential threats.

I have to say, the immune-system theory of aging is an elegant one. It has persuaded more than a few of my colleagues to assert with confidence that cranking up immunity can, in essence, turn back the clock. Our immune systems do get weaker with age. Older people do get cancer and infections more than young people. It doesn't take a huge leap of logic to surmise that strengthening immunity may in fact extend our lives.

Once again, however, interesting evidence isn't the same as proof, but this hasn't stopped the anti-aging specialists from giving it a shot—literally. In the last few years, an increasing number of patients who visit anti-aging clinics have been given injections of thymosin or other "glandulars." The idea is that increasing levels of these hormones will increase levels of T cells and so boost immunity and enhance the body's resistance to infections, cancer, or other threats. *But there is clear evidence, dating all the way back to the 1950s, that injections of thymosin or thymic cells have no measurable effect whatsoever on boosting the immune system.* And there's *no* evidence whatsoever that we can lengthen life or even ward off future diseases with these immune-boosting strategies.

Melatonin

Or consider the hype surrounding melatonin, a hormone that's been touted as an anti-aging immune enhancer. Produced by the pineal gland, melatonin appears to play a key role in regulating our internal clocks and promoting healthful sleep-wake cycles. More recently, we've learned from animal studies that high levels of melatonin increase levels of protective T cells. Melatonin also appears to have strong antioxidant capabilities. It may, in fact, be even more potent than vitamin E.

Melatonin is among the best-selling supplements in the United States, and it's widely promoted by physicians who are convinced that its *alleged* ability to enhance immunity can slow the aging process. Their evidence? A few studies that found that melatonin levels decline with age, and a single animal study that showed that low melatonin was linked to rapid aging.

I admit, these preliminary studies are intriguing. Were I involved in aging research, I'd certainly take a long look at melatonin as well as thymosin. But recommend them to my patients? Not a chance. So far, no one has come close to proving that melatonin (or other so-called immune enhancers, such as echinacea) has any long-term effects in humans. They certainly haven't been shown to extend life.

Maybe the immune system doesn't play a key role in the aging process after all. Maybe we just haven't stumbled on the right ways to make it stronger. In either case, there's no good evidence that tinkering with the immune system will help any of us live longer than we currently do. From what we can tell, in fact, the normal declines in immunity that occur with age are rarely severe enough to cause much harm. Yes, older people get more infections, and yes, they're more likely to get cancer. But these are hardly the only things that kill us in our later years. The body's immune system remains sufficiently robust throughout life to quell most of the threats it's designed to target. Aging has less of an impact on immunity than common lifestyle factors, such as malnutrition, smoking, or a lack of exercise.

I'm sure that in the years to come, as we learn more about how the immune system functions, we will develop treatments that will make us better able to withstand assaults from microorganisms as well as cancer. It's even possible that we'll identify immune deficiencies that shorten our average life spans. But that's a long way off. I don't hesitate to advise my patients to stay away from any treatment that's solely designed to enhance immunity as part of a life-extending regimen. The evidence just isn't there.

Correcting Hormonal Deficiencies

Nearly all of the body's hormones decline with age. The loss of estrogen in women after menopause is the most dramatic example. To a lesser extent, we also have declines in testosterone as well as hormones from the pituitary and thyroid glands. We know that many of the features of aging—lower energy and reductions in bone and muscle strength, to name just a few—can sometimes be explained by declining hormone levels. This has created the hope that routine hormone replacement might be the key to a longer as well as a healthier life. Indeed, physicians in anti-aging clinics may spend as much time checking for hormone deficiencies as they do looking at more conventional measures of health, such as cholesterol and blood pressure.

There are certainly times when deficiencies of key hormones can cause all sorts of problems. Giving supplemental hormones in these cases makes good sense. But what about giving hormones when a frank deficiency hasn't been identified? That's when things get more questionable—and a lot more controversial.

The Estrogen Question

Estrogen replacement is a perfect example of what can go wrong when doctors take limited knowledge and apply it to millions of patients. There's no question that estrogen deficiency in women is linked to many of the negative features of getting older. Menopause isn't a disease, but it is the time when estrogen levels fall and women start to experience bone loss, declines in libido and energy levels, and other symptoms.

Given the clear risks of low estrogen, it's hardly surprising that doctors handed it out like candy. Now, everything's changed. A large recent study found that estrogen replacement increased the risk of heart attack, blood clots, migraines, and a variety of cancers. Estrogen replacement will continue to be used in some cases, but I don't think you'll hear anyone touting it as a "treatment" for old age.

Growth Hormones

That's not the case with growth hormone. Many practitioners now endorse it great enthusiasm, and I have to say, it's a particularly attractive anti-aging candidate. Quite a few years ago, Dr. Daniel Rudman, one of the truly outstanding geriatric researchers, looked at a large number of frail, malnourished, elderly men. He found that many of them had low levels of growth hormone. When he gave them supplemental hormone injections, the improvements were dramatic. Their nutritional status returned to normal. They were stronger and more independent. Many of them, who seemed destined to spend their remaining time in nursing homes, were suddenly able to live on their own. The media, quite justifiably, was all over the study. CNN, in an excess of hyperbole, touted Dr. Rudman's findings as the "discovery of the Fountain of Youth."

Growth hormone is remarkable stuff. It's clearly indicated in those with frank deficiencies. Even in those with normal levels, supplemental doses promote an increase in energy and strength, which has made it one of the most popular of the illegal drugs used by professional athletes. But does it have any effect on the aging process? Not from what we can tell. Levels of growth hormone do decline with age, but they rarely decline so much that this causes much of a problem. There's no justification for giving it to normal people. Indeed, giving growth hormone to people who aren't deficient can cause all sorts of nasty complications, such as excessive bone growth in the face and hands, an increase in brain pressure, and even memory loss.

DHEA

Another hormone that's gotten a great deal of attention is DHEA, or dehydroepiandrosterone. It's a precursor hormone, one that's used by the body in the manufacture of estrogen, testosterone, and other hormones. It's an easy hormone to measure in the blood, and studies clearly show that levels decline with age. It's been suggested that raising levels of DHEA with supplementation can improve immunity, reduce free radical damage, and, possibly, extend life. It's available over the counter, and physicians who make their livings touting longevity treatments recommend it for just about everyone.

So far, nearly everything we know about DHEA comes from animal studies. Some of the findings have been provocative. It acts as an antioxidant by stimulating the production of superoxide dismutase. Mice given DHEA have lower blood sugar, better immune function, and less inflammation. Based on these studies alone, DHEA clearly deserves more research. But few good studies so far have been done in people, and the findings were less than overwhelming. One study found that elderly women who took DHEA did have slight gains in bone mass, along with increases in estrogen and testosterone. The increases were hardly significant, however, and the promising benefits that appeared in animal studies—better immunity, improvements in memory, and greater muscle size and strength—were not seen.

Given the paucity of evidence, I can't figure out why any reputable physician would recommend DHEA for generally healthy patients. It does appear to reduce side effects in women who are undergoing cortisol replacement therapy. DHEA also appears to make the tetanus vaccine work more efficiently in the elderly. Apart from this, it doesn't seem to have any practical benefits. Of course, this may change as we learn more about it. For now, we simply can't say that declines in DHEA have any practical impact. For all we know, lower levels may have beneficial rather than negative effects.

Testosterone

A lot of attention has been given to testosterone over the last few years. Between 10 and 15% of men ages 80 and older show declines in testosterone. It's been suggested that even slight declines in testosterone may cause weakness, fatigue, a loss of muscle mass, erectile dysfunction, and other age-related problems. Now some anti-aging doctors are giving testosterone to older men with the same abandon that physicians used to prescribe estrogen for women.

Should some men be given testosterone? Of course. Should it be used routinely? Hardly. Most men don't experience significant testosterone declines even in their later years. There's no evidence at all that modest reductions in testosterone have any effect on libido, strength, or anything else. A man who is truly deficient in testosterone will benefit from supplementation. A man whose testosterone levels have only dipped slightly will not. Yet testosterone is currently the drug of choice in the anti-aging community. It's being given by injection (cheap), patch (expensive), or creams and gels (very expensive) to thousands of men who have no need for it. These men will get bigger muscles, and it's theoretically possible that they might notice a slight increase in energy. They certainly won't live any longer than men who don't take it. Indeed, they might not live *as* long: Giving supplemental testosterone to men who aren't deficient can significantly increase the risk of heart disease.

Excess testosterone can also cause profound mood changes, including episodes of rage and violence.

So hormones aren't exactly the Fountain of Youth. Testosterone, along with growth hormone, DHEA, or other supplemental hormones, are helpful for those with clearly indicated medical problems. There's no evidence whatsoever that normal people will benefit from taking them. They won't live longer. They won't have more energy. They won't have stronger cells, better immunity, or more robust organ function. It may turn out that there are some real anti-aging approaches out there, but hormone replacement, from what I can see, isn't among them.

Genetic Manipulation

Thanks to the Human Genome Project, we now know the location of every gene on our 26 chromosomes—and our ability to understand life, disease, and aging has never been better. Of all of the anti-aging strategies that have been proposed (and largely abandoned) over the years, genetic manipulation shows the most promise. It won't happen in my lifetime, but I wouldn't be surprised if in the next 50 years scientists announce that they've finally discovered the secret to extending life.

There's a consensus among scientists that the lifespan of cells—and, by extension, the lifespans of we humans—are meticulously programmed by genes. We've already identified genes that seem to have the potential to expand longevity, along with the genes that shorten it. The science is still in its infancy, but as we learn more about how genes work, individually and collectively, we may finally unlock the mysteries of cellular aging.

Here's some of what we've learned so far. Laboratory studies have shown that cells can only divide a finite number of times. Once that number is reached, the cells no longer divide and eventually die, never to be replaced. There appear to be a number of genes in each cell that control this process—and with it, our maximum lifespans. It's too bad that there doesn't appear to be a single gene that controls how long cells live. If there were, it would be a relatively simple matter at some point to do some tinkering to change the way it functions. But there are multiple levels of genetic control in each cell. We're far from understanding how they work and how they interact with one another.

We've made some promising starts. A simple worm called *C. elegans*, for example, has a gene called clk-1. We've found that making the gene more active can increase the organism's lifespan by 50%. Were we to deliberately breed animals with the more active gene, we could create an entire line of long-lived organisms. Alternatively, we could snip out the gene, make copies, insert it in normal animals, and possibly extend their lives.

We've learned a great deal in the last few years about how genes regulate cellular aging. Every chromosome has a specialized structure on its end called a telomere. Each time cells divide, the telomere gets a little shorter. Eventually, it gets so short that the cell can no longer divide. A cell that can't divide has only a limited time to survive. We've also learned that an enzyme, telomerase, seems to prevent telomeres from getting shorter, thus prolonging cellular life. (The presence of telomerase in cancer cells may be what makes these cells immortal.) In the laboratory, it's possible to insert, or "transfect," telomerase into cells by attaching the gene to a benign virus. Once the virus carries its passenger into cells, it becomes a permanent part of the cell's DNA. The manipulated gene begins producing enough telomerase to prevent the telomere from getting shorter. Cells with more telomerase live longer and are able to divide many more times than cells without the enzyme. So it seems clear that genetic manipulation does have the potential to prolong the life of cells in a test tube. But extending this strategy to prolonging the lives of humans remains quite a challenge.

Researchers haven't focused specifically on using transfection to create long-lived cells (not to mention long-lived people). More important, to my way of thinking, is the possibility that we can use this approach—inserting, activating, or inhibiting genes—to cure a great number of diseases. This has already been done in children with severe immune system dysfunctions that forced them to live out their lives in sterile bubbles. I can certainly anticipate a time when the same approach might be used to reverse the loss of muscle that occurs with age, or even to help organs function longer.

At this point, though, we're nowhere near discovering how to genetically change an organism so that it's eternally young. Nor can we use this approach to expand longevity in people. But who knows what the future will bring? As we learn more about the aging process, on cellular as well as genetic levels, we very well may extend our normal lives to 160 years or even beyond.

THEORIES AREN'T TREATMENTS

I don't mean to apply that the scientific theories underlying all of the above "anti-aging" treatments are necessarily wrong. Quite the opposite. Many of them are intriguing and scientifically plausible. There's good evidence, for example, that the use of antioxidants may prevent or slow the progression of a number of age-related diseases. Growth hormone and testosterone clearly build muscle and improve strength in some people. But do either of these approaches slow or stop the aging process? Absolutely not. There's a world of difference between provocative and elegant research studies, which point us in new directions and may or may not lay the groundwork for practical applications, and the daily practice of clinical medicine. I'm afraid this distinction has been lost on some of these anti-aging physicians, who say that aging itself is a disease, and that we now have the tools to treat it—by increasing the activity within cells, for example, or slowing the rate of cellular death. Laboratory studies have indeed shown that some of these things are *theoretically* possible. What's true in theory, however, isn't always true—or at least immediately practical—in real life.

But I want to emphasize that some very important cellular research is emerging. There may come a time when we can use this information to reverse or stop the cellular damage that leads to aging and death. But before I sign off on any treatment for my patients, my family, or myself, I want to see the evidence. Have rigorous scientific studies shown that something works? What's the risk of side effects and complications? Anti-aging doctors have posed a lot of interesting hypotheses, but so far they haven't satisfactorily answered these questions. Until they do, I'm keeping my distance. So should you.

The search for eternal youth will always be an elusive, and perhaps impossible, goal. Yet there's so much we can do to move further in that direction. I already see it in my practice. Many of my patients come to see me not because they're sick, but because they want to stay healthy. It's a wise approach for all of us, especially those in their 50s and beyond who want to do everything they can to stay active and mentally and physically engaged. Personally, I'm much more interested in helping people have a quality life than an unduly long one. The medical students and residents I work with are always a little shocked when they overhear me tell my patients that my goal isn't to help them prolong their lives. Obviously, I do everything I can to treat diseases and keep them healthy, but longevity for longevity's sake isn't much of a goal. I'd rather see people live eventful, happy, high-quality lives—an attitude, by the way, that my older patients understand and relate to.

The baby boomers seem preoccupied with youth. The elderly know better. For them, quality beats quantity any day.

CHAPTER ELEVEN

"Well, when my time comes, I don't want any of that—things sticking out of my chest, respirators, tubes running up my nose....No thanks." —Larry, age 71

WHEN TO REFUSE THE "MIRACLES OF MEDICINE"

I wish I could reassure my patients that death, when it finally comes, will be merciful and quick. But the odds are against it. Only about 10% of deaths in older adults come quickly. Most of us will fall victim to prolonged, chronic illnesses, such as cancer, heart failure, and Alzheimer's disease—conditions that get progressively worse and rob us of our comfort and independence long before the end finally comes. I'm not surprised that most people are less afraid of death than of the suffering that precedes it. The ironic thing is that our medical system, in its determination to prolong life, has fostered the very circumstances that we fear most.

Our health care system views death as a failure—the failure of doctors and their latest high-tech, gee-whiz gizmos to preserve life at all costs. Our goal, always, is to keep patients alive for as long as possible, no matter how much they suffer. In the sterile, uncaring confines of intensive care units, with tubes in every orifice, patients are surrounded not by caring loved ones, but by efficient medical staff who deliver toxic drugs and administer the most painful and undignified treatments imaginable. Aggressive attempts at treatment and resuscitation make sense when survival is possible, but for terminal patients who will surely die in days or weeks, this refusal to bow to the inevitable can lead to horrifying deaths.

During my early medical training, I had the sad privilege of working with children who were dying from cancer. I learned more about life, strength, and dignity during those years than at any other time in my career. The children were the strong ones, the ones who brought a sense of calm and support to their frantic families. They approached death with an understanding and grace that I've rarely encountered in adults. Since then, I've made it a priority to help patients die with respect, peace, and comfort. Now, more than ever, I believe that a good death means a better life. The way we leave this earth has a profound impact on our lives, as well on the lives of those who live on and hold us in their memories.

POINTLESS HEROIC EFFORTS

One of my patients, a man with advanced Alzheimer's disease who had lost control over most of his bodily functions and no longer recognized his family, was clearly at the end of his life. His family understood that his condition was terminal, and they decided to keep him at home until the end.

But their plans for a natural, loving death for their father completely fell apart on the night when he aspirated food into his lungs, a common occurrence in the old and sick. His breathing became labored, and within a few hours he was completely unresponsive. The family panicked and called 911. The man was rushed by ambulance to the nearest emergency room.

Doctors unfamiliar with his condition and ignorant of his wishes did exactly what they were trained to do. They inserted a tube in his trachea to begin artificial respiration, and immediately transferred him to an intensive care unit (ICU). He was given antibiotics and intravenous fluids. A feeding tube was passed through his nose into his stomach. They kept him alive, all right, but he never regained consciousness. After six days of this pointless torment, the family, all but ignored by the hospital doctors, called and begged me to do something. I went to the hospital and met with the doctors, who admitted they'd known from the beginning that the man wasn't going to recover. The tubes were removed, he was transferred to a regular hospital ward and then to an inpatient hospice program, where he died peacefully five days later.

Why treat a patient so aggressively when he's obviously at the end of life? His doctors, had they taken the time to review his medical history, talk to the family, and question the very essence of their medical training, would have recognized the futility of their efforts. Yet their instincts told them to be as aggressive as possible. The man could have been allowed to die peacefully and naturally. Instead, he was needlessly tormented for days, and the family went through the kind of hell I wouldn't wish on anyone. And to what end?

Less than 100 years ago, nearly everyone died at home. Today, about 85% of deaths occur in hospitals or nursing homes. Families are no longer the primary caretakers. That role has been turned over to doctors and other health care professionals. The impersonal nature of institutional care, along with the usual time pressures and budget constraints, mean that the emotional and physical needs of the dying are increasingly overlooked.

An important research project, The Study to Understand Prognoses and Preferences for Outcomes and Risks of Treatments, illustrates just how bad end-of-life care can be. The study followed about 4000 patients from the time of their initial hospitalization until their death. Most of the family members surveyed felt that their loved ones suffered excessive and needless pain. About a quarter reported that their loved ones suffered from intense feelings of isolation and abandonment. Family members overwhelmingly reported that it was almost impossible for them to get clear explanations from physicians, or reassurances that their loved ones weren't suffering.

This survey, along with the impressions I've formed over decades of treating older patients, strongly suggests that ICUs are the worst possible places for dying patients. ICUs are busy, impersonal, and frantic. Patients get everything they need to survive and nothing that they need to *live*. There's no peace and quiet. Family members, when they're even allowed inside, are intimidated and constrained. Patients are continually being monitored, poked, and prodded. For those who are terminal, intensive care units almost guarantee that their final days or weeks will be filled with turmoil and pain, and wholly lacking in compassion, sensitivity, and comfort.

I recently learned that 27% of Medicare dollars go to acute, end-of-life care. What a tragic waste. The last thing terminal patients need is heroic medical efforts—efforts that can't possibly keep them alive, but only fill their final days with distress. Our medical system is the best in the world at treating disease, but it's pure arrogance to think we can deny death.

DYING A "GOOD DEATH"

I think the example above amply illustrates the unnecessary tragedy of a "bad death." Is there such a thing as a "good death"? I think there is.

One of my patients, who was living in an assisted living center, had a massive stroke. She had no chance of recovery, the neurosurgeon told her family. Even if doctors pulled out all the stops, and she somehow managed to survive, she was almost certain to remain in a vegetative state. Despite the poor prognosis, the surgeon and other doctors were still leaning toward surgery and other heroic measures to pull her through. To their credit, they took the time to discuss the pros and cons of treatment with the family. The family, of course, was conflicted: If they asked the doctors to do nothing, their mother would die. If they insisted on treatment, they would be ignoring their mother's wishes. She had made it quite clear that she didn't want heroic procedures to save her life. More than once she had expressed her dread of someday living as a vegetable in a nursing home.

The family decided against treatment. Their mother, they instructed, should be given comfort care only. She stayed in the hospital for two days, then was transferred to an inpatient hospice unit. Her relatives surrounded her bed with family pictures. They played her favorite music, and they stayed with her, in shifts, around the clock. There were no intravenous feedings, no invasive procedures. Their mother slept the whole time. After four days her blood pressure began to fall. Her heart beat became irregular. When she finally stopped breathing, her family was there, praying beside the bed. It was a good, natural death.

THE CRUELEST CARE

The American Medical Association has noted that only a handful of medical schools require courses in death and dying. Even residency programs in oncology and geriatrics rarely require formal training in treating the dying. This is starting to change, but most doctors are still woefully ignorant of this important part of medicine. Doctors practice what they know. This explains, I think, why they tend to recommend aggressive treatments for patients who can't possibly benefit. All of their training tells them that doing something is almost always better than doing nothing—even when that "something" can only prolong agony without improving or extending life.

This happens a lot with cancer patients. Cancer is a horrifying disease, one that can strike in the prime of life. It's almost unbearable for doctors, and for patients and their families, to even consider standing back and letting the disease run its course, even when there are no useful treatments. We tend to view cancer as this evil thing that grows inside us, one that must be fought at all cost. The "good fight," as it's called, is seen as positive and heroic. The reality, however, is that there are times when prolonging life means prolonging almost unspeakable suffering.

The Pros and Cons of Chemotherapy

Obviously, many cancers are worth fighting. We've taken enormous strides in the last 50 years. Cancers that were invariably fatal just a few decades ago can now be successfully treated with surgery, radiation, or chemotherapy. With early diagnosis, we cure many cases of leukemia and lymphoma. The same is true of cancers of the testicle, breast, uterus, cervix, and colon. Even many lung cancers can be cured when they're caught early enough. Even when a cure isn't possible, treatments such as chemotherapy and blood marrow transplants can shrink tumors and dramatically prolong life. The treatments may exact a heavy toll, but that's more than justified when the benefits are so dramatic.

Patients with advanced cancer, however, are routinely bombarded with near-lethal doses of radiation and drugs, even when oncologists acknowledge that the treatments are unlikely to help. It's hard for any of us to give up the fight, even when the outcome is all but guaranteed.

Patients can suffer tremendously, and needlessly, in their final months of life.

My heart still breaks when I remember one of my former patients, a 71-year-old woman with multiple myeloma, a particularly aggressive form of cancer. For nine months, she was given the most aggressive treatments available. She had many courses of chemotherapy, and a painful bone marrow transplant. After each grueling treatment, she heard the same story—the cancer wasn't responding. But the doctors, unwilling to admit defeat, kept trying. I'd like to say that their unflagging efforts were noble, that it's better to offer something, however slim the prospects, than to give up and quit. But there was a human being on the receiving end of all their efforts, and their treatments were making her life a living hell. That's not noble. It's wrong and uncaring, even cruel.

For nine long months, the poor woman was in severe pain. She couldn't walk or use the toilet without assistance. She had no appetite and lost more than 50 pounds. She was sick, frail, and tired—and still her doctors wouldn't give up. Her oncologist even advised her to undergo high-dose treatment with Cytoxan, a chemotherapeutic drug. This was truly grasping at straws. There's no evidence that Cytoxan can be effective in cases like this, and it would surely make her suffering worse. This is when the woman finally put a stop to it all—something her doctors should have had the courage and wisdom to do months before. "No more," she told them. "Please let me die in peace." She returned home and died five days later.

It's a tragic story, one that's repeated thousands of times every year. Not one of the doctors stepped back to really consider the consequences of the treatments. The poor woman was terrified, but received little attention or comfort from the doctors. She wasn't offered counseling. She suffered grievously from side effects, yet little effort was made to resolve them. Her doctors were so focused on battling the cancer that they pretty much forgot the suffering human being on the other end.

Don't get me wrong. I do believe that people have the right, even the duty, to do everything possible to save their lives. If there's a chance of a cure, or at least a significant lengthening of life, go for it. And I applaud the doctors who can make it happen. But I don't believe in promoting false hope. And I definitely don't believe in tormenting patients unnecessarily. There are times when aggressive treatments can only be said to extend suffering, not life.

There is no evidence, for example, that chemotherapy can prolong life in patients with a colon cancer that has spread beyond the bowel to the liver or other organs. Initial treatment with a chemotherapeutic drug called 5-FU is often used because in very rare cases it may shrink tumors slightly. But the drug is almost certain to be useless when a tumor has returned. Chemotherapy in these cases makes no sense at all, and side effects from the treatments can significantly degrade a patient's quality of life. I think that many patients, were someone to take the time to clearly explain the stark realities, would choose to forgo treatment. Yet doctors don't always tell the whole story. They might tell patients, for example, that the treatment has a 20% chance of shrinking the tumor, and a 1 in 100 chance of prolonging life. These dismal odds must seem better than nothing to patients fighting for their lives, but they're really not. Choosing a treatment with 1 in 100 odds is almost like praying for a miracle. People who undergo chemotherapy in these cases are unlikely to live any longer than those who don't get treatment, and their daily suffering from the treatments will be so severe that their remaining time can hardly be called living.

I strongly feel that patients with incurable diseases have the right to live their final weeks or months without unnecessary medical intervention.

Weighing the Balance: Will Chemo Help?

There are times when aggressive, end-of-life treatments are worth their weight in gold, even when a cure isn't possible: When they help patients live their final days free of pain and suffering. Radiation and chemotherapy are commonly used to temporarily shrink tumors and reduce painful symptoms. There will certainly be side effects, but they may be much less severe than pain from the disease itself.

When I see patients with terminal illnesses who are being advised to undergo aggressive, end-of-life treatments, I advise them to ask their oncologists or other doctors the following questions:

Will the treatment relieve symptoms? This is a common indication for chemotherapy and radiotherapy. For example, chemotherapy can reduce bone pain caused by many leukemias and lymphomas, even when a cure isn't possible. Chemotherapy can also reduce pain caused by prostate cancer.

Will the treatment prolong life? For recurrent cancers, this is very unlikely. Unless the treatment provides other benefits, like easing pain, think long and hard before agreeing to it.

What are the potential side effects, and how serious are they likely to be? You might decide you can live with severe side effects if the benefits are large enough. But if the treatment odds are very much against you, you have to wonder if it's worth going through it.

Will a treatment help others even if it's unlikely to help you? Many patients decide to go ahead with unproven therapies even when they know that their personal odds aren't very good. They do it because researchers can gain a great deal of knowledge that will help them treat future patients, and patients may find the thought of their own impending deaths more bearable when they know they've helped others. It's always possible, of course, that new, experimental treatments may turn out to be valuable for patients, as well. Participation in a well-designed clinical trial, conducted by a reputable cancer treatment specialist, provides access to state-of-the-art treatments and the latest breakthroughs. Tell your doctor if you'd like to participate in a peer-reviewed, federally funded research project that has received approval by the Institutional Review Board of an academic medical center. The review board ensures that studies are ethical, that patients fully understand the potential risks and benefits, and that there is clear value in participating.

DYING WITH COMFORT

Years ago, doctors referred to pneumonia as an "old man's best friend." Most people with terminal illnesses ultimately die of infections, and pneumonia was one of the main ones. Without treatment, pneumonia causes a progressive loss of consciousness and a gradual decline that eventually leads to death. It's a comfortable and painless way to die— and perhaps a great relief from the long-lasting agony of cancer and other terminal illnesses.

Today, of course, few doctors would welcome pneumonia in their terminally ill patients. I've seen people with end-stage cancer rushed into the emergency room, threaded with intravenous lines and flooded with antibiotics and fluids to bring them back to "health," even though their doctors know that they have, at most, a few days or weeks to live. Rather than being allowed to die naturally, surrounded by family and friends, these poor souls spend their final hours in intensive care units. I can't imagine a worse way to die—without comfort, without familiar faces, and without the comforts of home. And for what?

I hope that in the years to come, our health care system will finally come to terms with the inevitability of death. We all die, after all. It can't be postponed indefinitely. Death is always a loss, but it doesn't have to be preceded by prolonged and needless pain. We must learn to respect death as much as we do the miracle of life. There have been some promising steps in this direction. Nearly every hospital now offers hospice programs along with sophisticated palliative care.

Hospice and Palliative Care

Hospice, in case you're not familiar it, means caring for patients for whom there's no hope of recovery. Once patients are admitted to hospice programs—they include inpatient facilities as well as outpatient services and home visits—the goal is to help them live their final days without pain. Cure isn't on the agenda. People are encouraged to live their lives as fully as they're able, and then to die naturally when the time comes. They won't be rushed to the hospital because of pneumonia. Nature is allowed to take its course.

Hospice was initially developed to care for dying cancer patients, but it's now offered to anyone with a terminal illness. Many AIDS patients, for example, receive end-of-life care in hospice programs. So do older adults with end-stage Alzheimer's or heart disease.

The goal of both hospice and palliative care is to enable people to fully enjoy their remaining lives, without unnecessary or invasive treatments. Many hospice programs encourage patients to remain at home until the very end. Providing hospice care requires a committed team of medical professionals—doctors, nurses, pastors, social workers, and so on—who try to address every aspect of patients' lives, from their physical comfort to their spiritual, emotional, and mental health. They are all well trained in comfort care, and they do everything they can to help patients live comfortably, with a minimum of fear and pain.

Physician-Assisted Suicide

A palliative care team does a great deal to make life bearable. One of the main jobs of these teams is to give terminally ill patients the strength to carry on. Over the years, many of my patients have almost begged me to help them die. Physician-assisted suicide is one of the most difficult issues facing our society today. While I believe strongly that unnecessary prolongation of life is both cruel and uncaring, hastening death is something that should be, when patients receive appropriate pain relief and psychological support, totally unnecessary.

Some time back, one of my patients, a man in his late 80s with advanced colon cancer, stated in no uncertain terms that he wanted to end the suffering. He'd had a good life, he said, and he was blessed with a supportive and loving family. He was ready to die. "Will you help me end it?" he asked. Although I hadn't been involved in his cancer treatments, I had spent a great deal of time with him before his illness. I was certainly sympathetic to his request, and the thought did cross my mind that I could help him escape his suffering. I wasn't convinced, however, that suicide was the way to do it. I suspected that he was severely depressed—not only by impending death, but also by pain; it's been well established that the vast majority of cancer patients don't get anywhere near the pain relief they need. It was also likely that he was suffering fatigue due to anemia, a common side effect of chemotherapy. From what he told me, his doctors weren't all that interested in discussing his "aches and pains." They were sure aggressive about treating the cancer, but they were doing a terrible job of treating him.

I strongly encouraged him to have a frank talk with one of his oncologists, a woman I knew was blessed with an uncommon degree of empathy and patience. He made the appointment, and when I saw him again a few weeks later, he was a lot more upbeat. The doctor had switched him to more effective pain medications. She took care of the anemia, and also prescribed antidepressants. At the same time, she put him in touch with a behavioral medicine specialist—a psychotherapist who helped him find ways to cope with his imminent death—and encouraged him to meet with his minister for counseling. The man told me that suicide, for the time being, wasn't a direction he was going to take. He had some good months ahead of him, and he wanted to spend as much of the time as he could with his family and his wide circle of friends.

The Right to Pain Relief

A point that needs emphasizing is that it's almost always possible to reduce or eliminate discomfort caused by cancer and other terminal illnesses. It has to be done because patients who are grievously ill have enough on their plates as it is. Active, compassionate care does more than make the end of life bearable. It allows patients and their families to find meaning in their final weeks or months together. Dying can be a time for closeness, for providing reassurances, for saying goodbye. But this is only possible when discomfort from diseases or treatments is kept under tight control.

Unfortunately, this is done less often than you might think. The same doctors who will use every technique at their disposal to fight a disease are often sadly neglectful of the symptoms. Research has shown, for example, that more than 60% of cancer patients get inadequate pain relief. This issue has reached such a crisis point that more and more doctors are getting sued for not treating pain the way they should. In some states, in fact, giving inadequate levels of pain medication can lead to censure by state medical boards.

While many patients can control pain with over-the-counter analgesics or codeine in the early stages of their illnesses, morphine is clearly the treatment of choice when milder analgesics don't work. Physicians are often reluctant to prescribe morphine, and patients are unwilling to take it, because of the fear of addiction. This drives me nuts! A patient who is dying has nothing to fear from addiction and everything to fear from pain. Morphine works better than anything else, and patients should get all they need to be comfortable.

The Right to Forgo Nourishment

I'd like to make a final point about end-of-life care, one that often gets overlooked. Lost appetite, or anorexia, occurs with virtually every terminal illness, from cancer to Alzheimer's disease. I can't tell you how many times family members have said to me, "My mom"—or dad, husband, or wife—"refuses to eat and she keeps getting weaker. What can we do to make her eat?"

Giving food is one of the ways in which family members show their love and concern. We have this need to nurture, and it can become quite a sticking point. The person who is sick may not want to eat, and the family keeps pushing the issue. Watching a loved one wasting away invariably causes guilt and a very hopeless feeling. It's not surprising that doctors, with the encouragement of family members, often prescribe appetite-stimulating drugs, or even go so far as to insist on force-feeding. This type of artificial feeding does work, and it can certainly correct any nutritional deficiencies that may be present. Still, it's a miserable experience for all concerned.

I can think of a few circumstances when pushing food on someone who doesn't want to eat makes good medical sense. A cancer patient who's expected to live at least six months, for example, will benefit from getting adequate levels of nutrition. Six months in these circumstances is a long time, and it doesn't make sense for someone to waste away and lose strength and energy prematurely. The combination of an improved diet and regular exercise or physical therapy can result in quite an improvement.

One of my patients developed severe anorexia after surgery for lung cancer. His lack of appetite resulted in deficiencies of essential nutrients, among them zinc and vitamin A—nutrients that are necessary to promote normal appetite. He got locked in a vicious cycle: A lack of appetite caused by the illness resulted in malnutrition that further reduced his appetite. I didn't hesitate to prescribe appetite stimulants, along with nasogastric feeding for three weeks. This regimen, along with physical therapy, brought him back to normal in six weeks. He gained weight, his strength improved, and he was able to take care of himself without assistance.

But what about those who don't have long to live? The key issue, remember, is comfort. People who are dying deserve to live out their final days without unnecessary strife or discomfort. A lack of interest in food, and the resulting wasting away, is a natural progression of many diseases. It's almost as though the body is saying, "No more, I want to rest." Forcing terminal patients to eat against their will, however loving the intentions, may prolong life unnecessarily and add to their suffering. Gradual weight loss and malnutrition, on the other hand, are painless. Frankly, it's a good way to die—and it makes sense toward the end of life when all of the body's reserves are spent. You can keep someone alive with force-feeding, but why would you want to in these circumstances?

I generally advise families to make food available and to gently encourage their loved ones to eat. Providing meals is one more way for families to spend loving time together. If the patient doesn't want to eat, so be it. As I mentioned, it's not a painful process. Patients don't feel hunger or even much thirst. They just gradually fade away.

MAKE YOUR WISHES KNOWN

Death and dying are uncomfortable topics. I think we all have a tendency to ignore death, to somehow pretend that it's not going to happen to us or to our loved ones. But it will, of course. The older I get, the more comfortable I've become with the inevitability of it all. The thing that really scares me isn't death, but the idea that I'll suffer. I'm hardly alone in this. A great many of my patients—those in their 80s or 90s, for whom death isn't an abstraction—say the same thing. They don't want to be a burden on their families. They don't want to lose their mental abilities or their independence. They don't want to be in pain or lose control of their bodies. Death, it's been said, is easy, but dying can be very hard. Our medical system can make it even harder. You don't have to let this happen.

My philosophy is simple: Give me end-of-life care, not end-of-life heroics. I don't want teams of doctors beating on my chest, shoving tubes down my throat, and pumping drugs in my veins to keep me alive when my will to live is gone. I advise everyone to do what I have done: Make your wishes known before you get ill. I've frequently told my wife that if I ever get a terminal illness without a reasonable hope for recovery, she's not to fight to keep me alive. If my heart stops, don't resuscitate me. If I can't eat, don't force-feed me. If I get an infection, don't flood my blood with antibiotics. Let death take me when the time is right.

And please, when it's my time to go, don't put me in the hospital. Let me die at home, in my own bed, surrounded by the family I love so dearly. If my illness is such that I can't stay at home, enroll me in a hospice unit, where I'll be cared for by people who will anticipate my physical, emotional, and spiritual needs. "Death with dignity." It's become a cliché, but I can't think of a nobler goal. No tubes, no monitors, no catheters. Nothing that will demean me or change the way that my loved ones remember me when I'm gone.

I sometimes wish that all of my medical colleagues had the opportunity to work with dying children, as I did so many years ago. Their predicaments were dire, yet they faced every day with brave acceptance, hoping for the best, but also prepared for the worst. Death, they knew, is a natural part of life. We can only fight it for so long.

As a physician caring for elderly patients, I do everything I can to assure not only a longer life, but a life that is of the highest possible quality. But when there's no more hope, when the body is finally spent, I know it's time to step aside. I could care less about the "good fight." We each of us deserve a natural, comfortable death—a "good death." It's a fitting end to a good life.

CHAPTER TWELVE

"I thought retirement would be great, but it's not. My wife says I get in her way at home, most of my buddies are still back in Ohio, and all the grandkids are in Seattle now. I'm just bored. And nobody wants to hire an old man. Besides, I don't know anything about computers."   —Charlie, age 66

DOCTOR DAVID'S PRESCRIPTIONS FOR LIFE

Consider some of the geniuses of our time, "doddering old geezers" like Picasso, Titian, Mattisse, and Rubenstein. Or the entrepreneur Sam Walton, who orchestrated much of Wal-Mart's expansion after his 50th birthday. Think about Benjamin Franklin, who invented bifocals at age 78, or Michael De Bakey, the brilliant cardiac surgeon who stayed active into his 90s. Grandma Moses, the famous folk artist, didn't begin to blossom until her later years. She took up embroidery in her late 60s, but gave it up at 78 because of severe arthritis. She cast around for something else to do, and discovered her true gift as a painter. She completed one of her most famous canvases, *Rainbow*, when she was 101.

In my practice I've been humbled and inspired time and time again by patients who, at 55 start a new career, at 64 begin training for a marathon, at 72 go into business with a new partner, or at 78 become an award-winning gardener. At least once a day, someone comes into my office and shows me and my staff, by God, what old age is capable of. These are the ones who overflow with optimism, curiosity, and over-the-top energy. They'll tackle anything. They might not move as fast as they used to, and they might forget your name on occasion, but they sure as hell aren't sitting back and watching the world go by. They hold nothing back, and life gives abundantly back to them.

And that's the key, I believe: Not holding back; taking life as it comes and giving it all you've got. I've watched thousands of my patients approach middle age with more than a little trepidation, only to go through a second "late-blooming" stage as they hit their stride and embrace their advancing age—wrinkles, aches, and all.

In the preceding chapters I've given you my own "rules" for breaking the rules of aging. Now it's your turn. I'm going to give you a final, gentle push to get you out the door and into some of the best years of your life.

CULTIVATE CREATIVITY

I still remember the classic Art Linkletter line, "Getting older is not for sissies." I think there's a lot of truth to that. Once we pass our 50th birthdays, all sorts of things start going downhill. We have less energy. Our knees and backs complain more than they used to. Loud parties seem less attractive than quiet evenings at home. We're faced with retirement, financial changes, and a future that may seem somewhat empty. We're also watching our parents enter their later years, sometimes in robust good health, sometimes in decline. We worry that we'll become decrepit like they are.

A good number of my patients, I'm sad to say, do more than worry. They give up. "I'm not as young as I used to be" becomes the excuse for missing new movies, abandoning weekly poker games, or skipping neighborhood events.

It's not that these are weak people. It's just that ours is such a youth-worshipping society. We're surrounded by subtle (and not-so-subtle) messages that older adults, the helpless fools, have nothing to offer the world at large. In a society that expects so little from the elderly, it's hardly surprising that some people internalize the message and demand little from themselves.

Most people, however, refuse to buy into the youth myth. Creative talents like Grandma Moses and Picasso are, of course, hardly the only ones who experienced late-life blossoming. Dr. Keith Simonton, a professor of psychology at the University of California, Davis, has noted that many people experience a sudden surge in creativity when they reach their 60s and 70s. It's as though all of the creative energy of a lifetime finally comes together in what Dr. Simonton calls the "swan-song effect." In an intriguing study, he compared the last works of famous composers to the work they did earlier in life. He found that the later compositions were briefer, more restrained, and simpler, yet with great aesthetic qualities that make them some of the composers' most treasured works.

Our lives do slow down at retirement—which, to my way of thinking, is a blessing, not a hindrance. The physical changes that start to crop up during this time do impose limitations, but that shouldn't stop anyone from exploring creativity, finding new adventures, giving back to society. The happiest retirees are the ones who are teachers, artists, advisors, leaders—the ones, in short, who are totally engaged. Here in Little Rock, Arkansas, where I live, a woman named Mary Pru has been a real inspiration. She suffers from postpolio syndrome, and by age 70, was no longer able to live alone. She now lives in a nursing home, but she's hardly at the end of the road. Indeed, the changes in her life seemed to unlock new talents. She learned to paint watercolors, and her work is sold in local galleries. She also writes poetry, and her work gives meaning to her life and the lives of those who share it.

So it's quite clear that creativity—what might be called the zest for life—does not decline in any significant way as we get older. Indeed, Dr. Gene D. Cohen, of the Center on Aging, Health and Humanities at George Washington University, has made a compelling case that people who fill their lives with stimulation and satisfaction, and who maintain the belief that they have something to contribute, are the ones more likely to live long and healthy lives. And the longer they live, the more they contribute.

KNOW WHEN "AGE-RELATED" DISABILITIES AREN'T

Some of us, of course, will lose the good health that's so essential to a meaningful life. But this happens a lot less often than you might think. A more likely scenario is that we get brainwashed into short-changing our own potential. When you're convinced that life is downhill after retirement, it's seductively easy to give in to "age-related" disabilities that are, in fact, nothing of the kind.

About three years ago, I met with a man who was frantically worried about his parents. His father couldn't remember anything, he told me. He stumbled when he walked, and lately he'd become agitated and disruptive. His mother, though healthy, was calling him at all hours to complain about her husband's behavior and to discuss their financial difficulties. The family home, where they'd lived for more than 50 years, was cluttered and almost filthy. "Growing old is just awful," the son said.

Old, it turned out, had nothing to do with it. When I examined his father some weeks later, I was prepared to find evidence of Alzheimer's disease or stroke, which would explain his erratic behavior. What I found instead was that he had a severe deficiency of vitamin B12, along with a drinking problem he'd managed to conceal from his family for who knows how long. The poor man wasn't sick because he was old. He was just sick. I pumped him full of supplemental vitamin B12, got him into counseling for his drinking, and enlisted the help of social worker to help the family make some adjustments that were clearly overdue, like selling their enormous house and moving into something smaller and easier to care for. Today they've living in a small condominium. They exercise daily, travel often, and spend a lot of time with their children and grandchildren. Their future, once on the point of collapse, is now looking bright.

Sometimes we're forced to adjust to circumstances that change at a dizzying pace. This happens throughout life, but it tends to accelerate as we get older. Retirement, the death of friends or a spouse, and the specter of declining health can be painful blows. It's not old age that drags us down, but circumstances over which we feel we have no control. People can recover and move on from almost anything, but only when they have the self-esteem—and the external support from friends, relatives, and doctors—to believe that they can.

THE SIDE EFFECTS OF SELF-ESTEEM

If I had to pick one quality that I wish I could prescribe like pills from a bottle, it would be self-esteem. Research has clearly shown that people with strong self-esteem live longer than those who don't. It also seems to be the key to high-energy, successful aging. Self-esteem doesn't magically appear (or disappear) after retirement. It's something you have to cultivate your entire life. How you feel about yourself in your 50s will strongly determine your quality of life at age 70. Similarly, high self-esteem at age 70 is likely to predict a longer, higher-quality life.

A fascinating, long-running study looked at two groups of people: graduates of Harvard University and residents of inner-city Boston. One of the study goals was to determine some of the parameters of success-ful aging. The researchers found that people in both groups who described themselves as happy lived longer than those who didn't. But the Harvard graduates, who were more likely to have higher incomes, more stable family lives, and higher-self esteem, clearly had the edge. By age 70, 23% of the Harvard graduates had died, compared with 37% of the inner-city group.

Positive Reinforcement

Our society's attitudes toward older adults inevitably color how they view themselves. My good friend and colleague, Dr. Jeanne Wei, decided to measure the impact of attitudes on aging. She divided study partici-pants into two groups. People in both groups were instructed to sit in front of a computer screen that flashed subliminal messages. The mes-sages to one group were highly negative. Words such as *senile, depend-ent, disease,* and *disabled* flashed across the screen. The other group got positive messages: *wise, astute, revered, respected,* and *accomplished.* She found that people exposed to the negative stereotypes had higher blood pressure and faster heart rates than those exposed to the positive mes-sages. They performed less well on a battery of mathematical and verbal challenges. Even their balance was affected. Before sitting in front of the computer screens, people in both groups took about 76 seconds to walk some 50 feet. After the test, the negative-message group took 79 seconds to walk the same distance, while the positive-message group did it in 68 seconds. Based on this and other studies, it seems clear that positive reinforcement, which is one of the main ways in which we achieve self-esteem, is an important factor in good health.

"You look marvelous!"

Not so long ago, one of my patients told me how terrible she felt. It caught me by surprise because this lady, who's in her 80s, is usually upbeat and confident. It turns out that her granddaughter, the little gem, had the gracious good manners to say, "You look like shit, Grandma." The poor lady was devastated. She spent the next few days worrying about her looks, her intelligence, and just about everything else. Indeed, she spent a good part of our visit complaining about her weight and how ugly she felt. All from one stupid comment.

You can see why I spend a lot of my time trying to make patients feel better—not just with medical treatments, but with a few kind words. It sounds trite, but I've seen the results too often to dismiss it. I tell everyone who comes into my office, man or woman, how well they look. I sincerely mean it. None of us looks or feels the same as we did in the blooms of our youths, but so what? We should be proud of who we are, gray hair, wrinkles, and all. My advice, sappy though it sounds, goes something like this: "Wake up, look in the mirror, and tell yourself how gorgeous you are." Helping people feel good about themselves, and giving them tips on maintaining a positive attitude, does as much for health as checking blood pressure or writing a prescription.

In virtually every culture but our own, old people are appreciated and respected. That's the message we should be putting out, one that's upbeat and uplifting, not all this negativity about aging. Let's face it, those who have reached their 70s, 80s, or 90s in reasonably good health have done extremely well. They deserve to feel good about it.

FIND JOY IN RETIREMENT

How I envy one of my close friends, who decided to retire in his mid-50s after a successful career. At first, a lot of us thought he was crazy. Retirement, after all, is what you do toward the end of your life when your energies are more or less spent. How was this young and vigorous man going to spend his days? How will any of us, when retirement comes, find meaning without the satisfactions that come from work and worldly accomplishments?

Judging from my friend's example, it's no problem at all. He's fortunate enough to have enough money to live well, so that's not a problem. His days are remarkably full. He volunteers for a number of groups. He offers his business expertise to those who need it. He travels, exercises, meets friends for lunch, and generally stays as busy as he ever was. The only difference is that he no longer works 60 to 80 hours a week in a high-stress job. The last time I saw him, he looked happy and fit as a fiddle. He's made retirement work. There's absolutely no reason why you can't do the same.

Plan ahead. I think the majority of older adults do very well in retirement, although the first year or two can present some rocky challenges. People who were intensely focused on their careers, often to the exclusion of their "real" lives, have the hardest time. They have to fill their days somehow, and this requires developing new interests and talents outside the workplace. One of my patients had a terrible time once he gave up control of the company he'd spent decades building. He's a take-charge kind of guy, and all of a sudden he had nothing to take charge of. He'd been so focused on his career that he had no outside interests—no hobbies, no sports, no friends. Without work, he felt empty and alone. Unlike my friend, who found great joy in retirement, this poor man struggled to get through each day.

Place value in things besides work. It's a risk that we, the baby boomers, would do well to be aware of. It's not that we work harder than our parents, but that we put so much emphasis on occupational success that we tend to forget all the other things that make life worth living. We might be able to buy fancy cars and expensive gadgets, but we're not developing the skills that we'll surely need later on. I hear so many people say, "I intend to work until the day I die." I suppose that's an admirable goal if you love your work, and if you're lucky enough to stay healthy right up to the end. For most of us, though, it's an unrealistic goal, and a lousy way to prepare for life's next transition. Work is good, no doubt about it. But there are so many other important things in life: grandchildren, travel, time with your spouse, and new challenges and tasks. It's a tragedy when people spend their lives so consumed by work that they can't see their way clear to a new life when the time comes. They're the ones for whom retirement threatens to be a burden rather than a precious time of opportunities.

Stay busy. A great deal of research has focused on the health effects of retirement. Some of the findings have been surprising. The mental health of most retirees is *better* than it was prior to retirement. Surveys show that most people find retirement to be a liberating time. They have less anxiety and stress, and they enjoy life more than they did during their working years. Obviously, this only applies to those who remain actively engaged in life. If your idea of retirement is watching the grass grow, you're going to have some long days ahead of you. Most people, of course, know better. In my practice, the healthiest patients are the ones who stay busy. They launch new careers, albeit careers with shorter hours and less stress than the ones they left behind. They take university classes, join gardening groups, get more serious about hobbies they always enjoyed but never had time for. Volunteering is a big deal in these age groups, and for good reason. The elderly are the most economically stable segment of our society, and they have both the time and expertise to give back to the world they made.

Make friends and maintain social networks. It's never enough to retreat into the bosom of family. Certainly, spending time with your spouse, children, and grandchildren is a good thing. But you also need to maintain strong social networks, if only to get out of the house and out of your spouse's hair! I encourage everyone to cultivate friendships, to stay in touch with acquaintances who may be drifting way. The more active you are in your community, the happier and more satisfied you're going to be. Definitely make children part of your life. I'm hardly alone in believing that one of the main responsibilities of older generations is to pass along their knowledge and experiences to the ones who follow. A recent study of older adults who participated in a foster grandparent program found that a whopping 97% felt that their work was not only important, but gave them great satisfaction.

Stay alert for depression—and treat it! One of the unspoken difficulties of the retirement years, and one that doesn't get anywhere near enough attention, is depression. It's a terrible problem for anyone, and it can be especially acute in the elderly. They've gone through major life changes that they may or may not be fully equipped to handle. They've left the careers that gave their lives meaning and purpose. Children may have scattered, and they've undoubtedly lost friends or loved ones. On top of all this, they're physiologically more prone to depression. They're less able to replenish supplies of noradrenalin and serotonin, brain chemicals that play a key role in regulating mood. Low levels of these chemicals can result in insomnia, fatigue, and other physical symptoms. Without treatment, depression can make the days seem empty and the future bleak.

As I mentioned before, high self-esteem and a positive attitude are critical components of both health and happiness. Any degree of depression, or even a pervading sense of glumness, has to be dealt with. Frankly, it's not all that hard to do. Anyone who's feeling down for more than a few weeks should definitely see a doctor. There are literally dozens of illnesses that can cause depression. Indeed, any condition that hurts or drags down your energy is going to affect your mood to some extent. Many common drugs, such as beta-blockers and tranquilizers, can trigger depression. So, of course, can excessive alcohol consumption. Treating the physical problems will often take care of the emotional issues at the same time.

I don't hesitate to recommend drug therapy for depression. The new generations of antidepressants, such as Prozac, Paxil, Zoloft, and Celexa, elevate serotonin levels in the brain. The drugs take about two weeks to work, but the results can be dramatic. They're especially effective when people also see a psychologist or counselor—someone who can help them understand the changes in their lives and develop more effective ways of dealing with them.

One final word about depression. Be on the lookout during the winter months. The days are shorter and there's less sunlight, which invariably makes depression worse. The holiday season can be particularly hard for the elderly. Instead of feeling joy, they may find themselves yearning for a time when life seemed better. A little reassurance, and a lot of time together, can go a long way.

EMBRACE SPIRITUALITY

A great many of my patients, in fact, perhaps most of them, have a deep and abiding belief in some higher power. Many of them are religious and attend services regularly. Others, less formal in their beliefs, embrace a sense of community and oneness with the world and the people around them. As a physician, my natural inclination is to focus mainly on the physical or psychological dimensions of patient care. But I've learned over the years to take my patients' spiritual leanings seriously. In fact, I added a new item to my standard questionnaire: "Is religion important in your life?" Apart from the fact that religion and spirituality can give people a great deal of comfort during difficult times, there's good evidence that people who cultivate their spiritual sides tend to be healthier than those who don't.

It's only in the last decade or so that researchers have taken a good look at the effects of prayer, meditation, and other religious or spiritual practices on long-term health. What they've found has been remarkable. One large study, for example, followed more than 5000 adults for 28 years. Researchers found that those who frequently attended religious services were 23% less likely to die during the study period than those who didn't attend services. Men who are religious have 35% less heart disease than those who aren't. People who participate in religious activities of all kinds have lower blood pressure and less risk of hospitalization than those who don't participate. Even those who are seriously ill—with cancer or AIDS, for example—seem to have a better quality of life when they incorporate some form of religion in their lives.

It doesn't seem to matter whether you go to service regularly, or even were raised in a religion tradition. Research has shown that it's not what people believe that influences their health, but the mere fact that they do believe. Embracing a higher power of any kind seems to be the answer to a longer and healthier life.

We're still not sure what it is about religious or spiritual beliefs that promotes good health. One theory is that activities such as prayer, meditation, and worship, and the embrace of positive emotions such as hope and love, cause a sharp reduction in hostility and anger—emotions that have clearly been shown to increase the risk of heart disease and other health threats. It's also likely that social interactions play a role. People who are active in their religious community or prayer groups spend time with like-minded people, which gives them sense of connectedness and belonging, qualities that have been clearly linked with longevity.

Put religion and spirituality aside for a moment. There's good evidence that merely avoiding stress and staying calm and tranquil provide exactly the same benefits as attending services or participating in a spiritual community. This is often the answer for those don't have a religious or spiritual bent. Indeed, research by Dr. Dean Ornish suggests that meditation is the single most important factor in reducing the risk of a second heart attack following an initial episode.

I don't think we'll ever know for sure how spirituality and prayer affect health. All we can say for sure is that they're clearly beneficial.

MAKE THE BEST OF THE BEST YEARS

But religious or not, what really matters is the whole bundle of attitudes with which you face life. Strong self-esteem and a positive mental attitude are undoubtedly as important as spiritual practices. Appreciating yourself and the world around you counts. So does remaining creative and mentally active throughout your life.

I wish it were possible to insert an emotional "cheat sheet" in people's brains, something they could refer to daily in the many years after retirement. So many of the stereotypical images of the postretirement years—depression, lack of energy, diminished creativity, and so on—are flat-out wrong, especially among those who do a few simple things:

Love yourself. The evidence is conclusive: Self-esteem is among the most powerful predictors of good health and a long life. Feel good about yourself. Appreciate your inner and outer beauty. Wake up every morning, stand naked in front of a mirror, and say, "You are gorgeous!"

Find the bright side, always. It's not always easy to have a positive attitude, but do your best. No matter how bad things get, you still have a lot to give the world.

Retirement isn't an end to anything. It's a beginning, so treat it that way. Get busy and stay busy. Life has to be full to have meaning.

Cultivate your creative side. Write, paint, restore old cars. You don't have to be good at it. You just have to enjoy it.

Stay close to your family. We are now the older ones. It's up to us to mentor our children and grandchildren, and to pass on the knowledge they'll need in time.

Get in touch with your spiritual side. At the very least, do whatever it takes to stay calm and peaceful. You'll not only feel better, you'll live longer.

There is nothing—and I mean nothing—that you can't do.

Play, create, have sex, travel. Enjoy life to the fullest.

What's age got to do with it?

INDEX